DISABILITY STUDIES

DISABILITY

INTERNATIONAL ASPECTS

DISABILITY STUDIES

Joav Merrick - Series Editor –

NATIONAL INSTITUTE OF CHILD HEALTH AND HUMAN DEVELOPMENT, MINISTRY OF SOCIAL AFFAIRS, JERUSALEM

Disability: International Aspects
Ariel Tenenbaum and Joav Merrick (Editors)
2020. ISBN. 978-1-53617-886-9 (Hardcover)
2020. ISBN. 978-1-53617-887-6 (e-book)

Pain Management Yearbook 2017
Joav Merrick (Editors)
2018. ISBN: 978-1-53613-693-7 (Hardcover)
2018. ISBN: 978-1-53613-694-4 (e-book)

Quality of Life and Intellectual Disability: Knowledge Application to other Social and Educational Challenges
Roy I. Brown and Rhonda M. Faragher (Editors)
2014. ISBN: 978-1-62948-264-4 (Hardcover)
2018. ISBN: 978-1-53613-063-8 (Softcover)
2014. ISBN: 978-1-62948-272-9 (e-book)

Parkinson's Disease: Awareness among Young Adults
Ronald Chow, Jaclyn Viehweger, Michael Borean, Drew Hollenberg, and Joav Merrick (Editors)
2017. ISBN: 978-1-53612-745-4 (Hardcover)
2018. ISBN: 978-1-53612-745-4 (Softcover)
2017. ISBN: 978-1-53612-746-1 (e-book)

Human Development: Equipping Minds with Cognitive Development
Carol T. Brown and Joav Merrick
2018. ISBN: 978-1-53613-053-9 (Softcover)
2018. ISBN: 978-1-53613-054-6 (e-book)

Autism Spectrum Disorder: Awareness among Young Adults
Ronald Chow, Jaclyn Viehweger, Joav Merrick (Editors)
2017. ISBN: 978-1-53612-730-0 (Hardcover)
2017. ISBN: 978-1-53612-731-7 (e-book)

Virtual Reality: Recent Advances in Virtual Rehabilitation System Design
Wendy Powell, Albert "Skip" Rizzo, Paul M. Sharkey and Joav Merrick
2017. ISBN: 978-1-53612-040-0 (Softcover)
2017. ISBN: 978-1-53612-061-5 (e-book)

Child Abuse: Children with Disabilities
Vincent J Palusci, Dena Nazer, Donald E Greydanus and Joav Merrick
2017. ISBN: 978-1-53612-035-6 (Hardcover)
2017. ISBN: 978-1-53612-056-1 (e-book)

Rehabilitation: Innovations and Challenges in the Use of Virtual Reality Technologies
Wendy Powell, Albert "Skip" Rizzo, Paul M. Sharkey and Joav Merrick, (Editors)
2017. ISBN: 978-1-53612-080-6 (Hardcover)
2017. ISBN: 978-1-53612-099-8 (e-book)

Virtual Reality: Recent Advances for Health and Wellbeing
Wendy Powell, Paul M Sharkey and Albert "Skip" Rizzo
2017. ISBN: 978-1-53612-454-5 (Softcover)
2017. ISBN: 978-1-53612-455-2 (e-book)

Pediatric Pain: Current Aspects
Hatim A. Omar, Dilip R. Patel, Donald E. Greydanus, and Joav Merrick (Editors)
2016. ISBN: 978-1-63485-505-1 (Hardcover)
2016. ISBN: 978-1-63485-537-2 (e-book)

Recent Advances on Using Virtual Reality Technologies for Rehabilitation
Paul M. Sharkey and Joav Merrick (Editors)
2016. ISBN: 978-1-63484-027-9 (Hardcover)
2015. ISBN: 978-1-63484-028-6 (e-book)

Technology, Rehabilitation and Empowerment of People with Special Needs
Lena Pareto, Paul M Sharkey and Joav Merrick (Editors)
2015. ISBN: 978-1-63482-713-3 (Hardcover)
2015. ISBN: 978-1-63482-737-9 (e-book)

Virtual Reality: Rehabilitation in Motor, Cognitive and Sensorial Disorders
Paul M. Sharkey and Joav Merrick (Editors)
2014. ISBN: 978-1-63321-773-7 (Hardcover)
2014. ISBN: 978-1-63321-787-4 (e-book)

Virtual Reality: People with Special Needs
Paul M. Sharkey and Joav Merrick (Editors)
2014. ISBN: 978-1-63321-729-4 (Hardcover)
2014. ISBN: 978-1-63321-734-8 (e-book)

Intellectual Disability: Some Current Issues
Joav Merrick, Donald E Greydanus and Dilip R. Patel (Editors)
2014. ISBN: 978-1-63321-855-0 (Hardcover)
2014. ISBN: 978-1-63321-867-3 (e-book)

From One Century to the Next: A History of Wrentham State School and the Institutional Model in Massachusetts
Ingrid Grenon
2014. ISBN: 978-1-63117-711-8 (Hardcover)
2014. ISBN: 978-1-63483-805-4 (Softcover)
2014. ISBN: 978-1-63117-712-5 (e-book)

Pain and the Elderly
Joav Merrick and Mimi M.Y. Tse
2013. ISBN: 978-1-62948-468-6 (Hardcover)
2013. ISBN: 978-1-62948-475-4 (e-book)

Pain: International Research in Pain Management
Joav Merrick, Patricia Schofield and Mohammed Morad (Editors)
2013. ISBN: 978-1-62948-423-5 (Hardcover)
2013. ISBN: 978-1-62948-435-8 (e-book)

Disability and Chronic Disease
Joav Merrick, Shoshana Aspler and Mohammed Morad (Editors)
2013. ISBN: 978-1-62948-288-0 (Hardcover)
2013. ISBN: 978-1-62948-307-8 (e-book)

Down Syndrome and Dementia. A Comprehensive and Historical Review
Vee P. Prasher
2012. ISBN: 978-1-62081-263-1 (Hardcover)
2012. ISBN: 978-1-62081-271-6 (e-book)

Rett Syndrome: Therapeutic Interventions
Meir Lotan and Joav Merrick (Editors)
2011. ISBN: 978-1-61728-614-8 (Hardcover)
2011. ISBN: 978-1-61728-080-1 (Softcover)
2011. ISBN: 978-1-61761-131-5 (e-book)

Pain Management Yearbook 2010
Joav Merrick (Editor)
2011. ISBN: 978-1-61209-972-9 (Hardcover)
2011. ISBN: 978-1-62808-255-5 (e-book)

Pain Management Yearbook 2009
Joav Merrick (Editor)
2011. ISBN: 978-1-61209-666-7 (Hardcover)
2011. ISBN: 978-1-62081-774-2 (e-book)

Pain. Brain Stimulation in the Treatment of Pain
Helena Knotkova, Ricardo Cruciani and Joav Merrick (Editors)
2011. ISBN: 978-1-60876-690-1 (Hardcover)
2011. ISBN: 978-1-61470-495-9 (e-book)

Neural Plasticity in Chronic Pain
Helena Knotkova, Ricardo A. Cruciani and Joav Merrick (Editors)
2011. ISBN: 978-1-61324-657-3 (Hardcover)
2011. ISBN: 978-1-62417-407-0 (e-book)

Disability from a Humanistic Perspective: Towards a Better Quality of Life
Shunit Reiter
2011. ISBN: 978-1-60456-412-9 (Hardcover)
2011. ISBN: 978-1-63117-654-8 (e-book)

Cancer in Children and Adults with Intellectual Disabilities: Current Research Aspects
Daniel Satgé and Joav Merrick (Editors)
2011. ISBN: 978-1-61761-856-7 (Hardcover)
2011. ISBN: 978-1-61122-187-9 (e-book)

Contemporary Issues in Intellectual Disabilities
V. P. Prasher
2010. ISBN: 978-1-61668-023-7 (Hardcover)
2010. ISBN: 978-1-61209-292-8 (e-book)

Disability Studies

Disability

International Aspects

Ariel Tenenbaum, MD
and
Joav Merrick, MD, MMedSci, DMSc
Editors

nova
Medicine & Health
New York

Library of Congress Cataloging-in-Publication Data

ISBN: 978-1-53617-886-9

Published by Nova Science Publishers, Inc. † New York

CONTENTS

INTRODUCTION

In: Disability: International Aspects
Editors: Ariel Tenenbaum et al.
ISBN: 978-1-53617-886-9

Chapter 1

IS DISABILITY RESEARCH SOMETHING IMPORTANT?

Ariel Tenenbaum[1-3], MD
and Joav Merrick[2-5,*], MD, MMedSci, DMSc
[1]Center for Children with Chronic Diseases and Down Syndrome Center Jerusalem, Israel
[2]Department of Pediatrics, Mt Scopus Campus, Hadassah Hebrew University Medical Center, Jerusalem, Israel
[3]National Institute of Child Health and Human Development, Jerusalem, Israel
[4]Kentucky Children's Hospital, University of Kentucky, Lexington, Kentucky, United States
[5]Center for Healthy Development, School of Public Health, Georgia State University, Atlanta, United States

---

* Corresponding Author: Professor Joav Merrick, MD, MMedSci, DMSc, Director, National Institute of Child Health and Human Development, Jerusalem, Israel. E-mail: jmerrick@zahav.net.il.

ABSTRACT

Disability research is important for the individual, the family, but certainly also for the society that has to adapt and facilitate an easier life and better service for this segment of our populations. For example research showed significant disparities in the prevalence of disability between urban and rural residents, which can guide society to provide better service. Epidemiology and survey research can be important tools for public health focus and intervention and guide policy makers to allocate budgets and service facilities and expertise. In this book we have gathered research on various aspects of disability from Malaysia, India, Ghana, Kenya, Portugal, Bangladesh, Thailand and Nigeria, which we hope will be of interest to the reader.

INTRODUCTION

You can ask yourself if disability research is important? Wherever we live or whatever we do or with whom we live, disability will always be something that will be part of us … if we want to know or even if we do not. With increasing age disability for sure will be something that we all will encounter. It can be age or it can be outside forces that will result in disability, like for example a traffic or any other accident.

CHILDREN

Developmental disability in childhood refers to a group of conditions that are the result of impairment in physical, learning, language, behavior or intellectual capacity (1). These conditions begin during the developmental period and may impact day-to-day functioning and often can last throughout life.

Some of these disabilities start already during pregnancy or in early childhood development caused by injury, infection, genetics or unknown or a mixture of factors. The "Study to explore early development" (SEED) is a multiyear study funded by the CDC. It is currently the largest study in the United States to help identify factors that may put children at risk for autism spectrum disorders and other developmental disabilities (2). Here are some of the examples of developmental disabilities (2):

- At least 25% of hearing loss among babies is due to maternal infections during pregnancy, such as cytomegalovirus (CMV) infection, complications after birth and head trauma.
- Some of the most common known causes of intellectual disability include fetal alcohol syndrome; genetic and chromosomal conditions, such as Down syndrome and fragile X syndrome and certain infections during pregnancy.
- Children who have a sibling with autism are at a higher risk of also having autism spectrum disorder.
- Low birthweight, premature birth, multiple birth, and infections during pregnancy are associated with an increased risk for many developmental disabilities.
- Untreated newborn jaundice (high levels of bilirubin during the first few days after birth) can cause a type of brain damage known as kernicterus. Children with kernicterus are more likely to have cerebral palsy, hearing and vision problems, and problems with their teeth. Early detection and treatment of newborn jaundice can prevent kernicterus (2).

Data from the US National Health Interview Survey 2014-2016 (3) showed an increase from 5.75% to 6.77% in the prevalence of children aged 3-17 years ever diagnosed with a developmental disability. The prevalence of diagnosed autism spectrum disorder and intellectual disability did not change significantly (2.24% to 2.76%). The prevalence of autism spectrum disorder, intellectual disability (1.10% to 1.14%), other developmental delay (3.57% to 4.55%) and any developmental disability (5.76% to 6.99%) was higher among boys compared with girls. The prevalence of any developmental disability was lower among Hispanic children compared with children in all other race and ethnicity groups.

Adults

Data from the United States 2016 Behavioral Risk Factor Surveillance System were analyzed for adult prevalence of disability and disability types by urban-rural county classification (4). The prevalence of having any disability, functional disability type, or multiple disabilities was lowest in large metropolitan centers and fringe metropolitan counties and highest in rural or non-core counties. After controlling for age, sex, race, ethnicity, education and federal poverty level, adults living in non-core counties were 9% more likely to report having any disability, 24% more likely to report having three or more disabilities and 7% (cognition) to 35% (hearing) more likely to report specific disability types than the adults living in large metropolitan centers.

Globally

Based on 2010 global population estimates, the World Health Organization (WHO) and the World Bank (5) estimated that more than a billion people live with some form of disability. This means about 15% of the population in the world, which is 5% higher than an earlier WHO estimate from the 1970s (5).

Conclusion

We think that disability research is important. The research is important for the individual, the family, but certainly also for the society that has to adapt and facilitate an easier life and better service for this segment of our populations. For example research from the United States (4) found significant disparities in the prevalence of disability between urban and rural residents with rural residents having the highest prevalence of disability (4). Such epidemiology and survey research can be important tools for public health focus and intervention and guide policy makers to allocate budgets and service facilities and expertise. In this book we have gathered research on various aspects of disability from Malaysia, India, Ghana, Kenya, Portugal, Bangladesh, Thailand and Nigeria, which we hope will be of interest to the reader.

REFERENCES

[1] Rubin IL, Merrick J, Gredanus DE, Patel DR, eds. Health care for people with intellectual and developmental disabilities across the lifespan. Cham, Switzerland: Springer International, 2016.

[2] CDC. Facts about developmental disabilities. URL: cdc.gov/ncbddd/developmentaldisabilities/facts.html.

[3] Zablotsky B, Black LI, Blumberg SJ. Estimated prevalence of children with diagnosed developmental disabilities in the United States, 2014-2016. NCHD Data Brief 2017;291.

[4] Zhao G, Okoro CA, Hsia J, Garvin WS, Town M. Prevalence of disability and disability types by urban-rural county classification-US 2016. Am J Prevent Med 2019;57(6):749-56.

[5] Thompson S. Disability prevalence and trends. URL: http://www.gsdrc.org/wp-content/uploads/2017/09/179-Disability-prevalence-and-trends.pdf.

SECTION ONE:
INTERNATIONAL ASPECTS OF DISABILITY

In: Disability: International Aspects
Editors: Ariel Tenenbaum et al.
ISBN: 978-1-53617-886-9

Chapter 2

PEOPLE WITH DISABILITIES: AN ANCIENT SOCIETY GOT IT RIGHT, BUT CAN WE?

Nor IA Razak**, MMedSc, BSc,
Nazirah Hasnan, PhD, MRehabMed, MBBS,
Ku ASI Putera, MSc, BSc,
Jayaletchumi Gunasagaran, Ms Orth, MBBS
and Tunku S Ahmad, FRCS, MBBS
National Orthopaedic Centre of Excellence for Research and Learning (NOCERAL), Department of Orthopaedic Surgery, Faculty of Medicine, University of Malaya, Kuala Lumpur, Malaysia, Department of Rehabilitation Medicine, Faculty of Medicine, University of Malaya, Kuala Lumpur, Malaysia and Institute of Health Systems Research, Ministry of Health, Selangor, Malaysia

* Corresponding Author: Nor IA Razak, MMedSc, BSc, Research Associate, National Orthopaedic Centre of Excellence for Research and Learning (NOCERAL), Department of Orthopaedic Surgery, Faculty of Medicine, University of Malaya, 50603 Kuala Lumpur, Malaysia. Email: zatirazak@um.edu.my.

ABSTRACT

Persons with disabilities of today often have difficulty reaching full career and social status, due to physical, functional, practical and psychological factors. The Lenggong Valley, in the state of Perak, Malaysia contains the 11,000 year old remains of a member of the Austramelenesoid family. He was tall, but had several abnormalities. He had a skeletal deformity of the upper limb. His elbow was held flexed, wrist extended and he had an abnormal left middle finger. He also had a scoliosis and a shorter left lower limb. It is estimated that he walked with a limp. However he is estimated to have died at the age of 40 to 45 years, twice the life expectancy of his time. Archeological findings indicated that he was buried as an important person in the tribe, possibly a Shaman. With his abnormalities, he was probably unable to hunt effectively, yet obviously given a more appropriate role to play and able to lead a long life of a respected person, being buried with full honours of his time. An ancient civilization was able to adapt roles so that a person with disabilities could use his unique abilities to contribute to society and lead a respected life, something present society could think about and learn from. If current society could help the disabled to achieve their full potential, everyone would stand to benefit.

INTRODUCTION

Persons with disability in the 21st century still face more frequent hardships with a greater impact then others (1). They are then less able to exercise rights, form their true or best "identity" (2) and reach their full potential both socially and also in their careers (3, 4). They are thus negatively discriminated against especially in rural underdeveloped societies (5).

The Lenggong Valley, in the state of Perak, Malaysia contains the remains of an extraordinary man. Named the Perak Man, he lived in the Paleolithic period and was a member of the Austramelenesoid family found in Australia, Indonesia, Papua New Guinea and Malaysia. His eleven thousand year old skeleton, the oldest complete skeleton to be found in South East Asia, tells an interesting story.

He was buried in a fetal position. His estimated height was approximately 154 cm. He had a long head and narrow face. His cranium, humerus, femur and tibia have similar traits and are morphologically linked with Australomelanesoid affinity, a race occupying the western part of Indonesia, now largely confined to east Indonesia, Melanesia and Australia.

THE PERAK MAN

Archeological excavations have been conducted by the Centre of Archeological Research, Malaysia, followed by multidisciplinary and scientific study of the skeletal remains. Cave drawings by local indigenous people have made the Lenggong Valley one of the icons of pre-historical times in its region. The Perak Man was discovered with only a few missing bones such as a metatarsal, and parts of the face, making him one of the earliest most-complete pre-historic human skeletons in Southeast Asia in its ancient times ranging from 10,000 – 11,000 years ago (6).

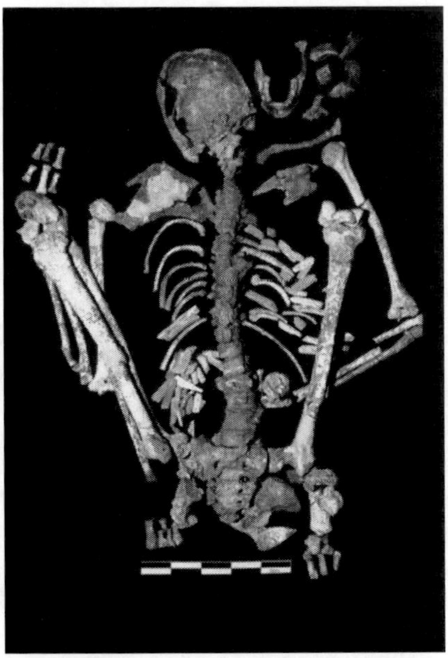

Figure 1. A full skeleton of Perak man.

The deformities

Physical examination of the skeleton was first conducted on-site and later followed by analyses in the geochronology laboratory. The statistical comparison of the biological distances, based on the dental and limb metric traits, suggested that the Perak Man was morphologically linked to the Australo-Melanesian. Detailed analyses of the remains showed that he was born with several abnormalities:

- The arm: He had a skeletal deformity of the left upper limb, which was markedly shorter than the right. His left elbow was held flexed and wrist extended. The shortening indicates that he could have had a congenital abnormality. The shafts of his left ulna and radius were shorter, abnormally thin and anteriorly curved (see Figure 1). With a form and posture like that, he could have suffered from a congenital neurological abnormality such as cerebral palsy or brachial plexus birth palsy or even polio.

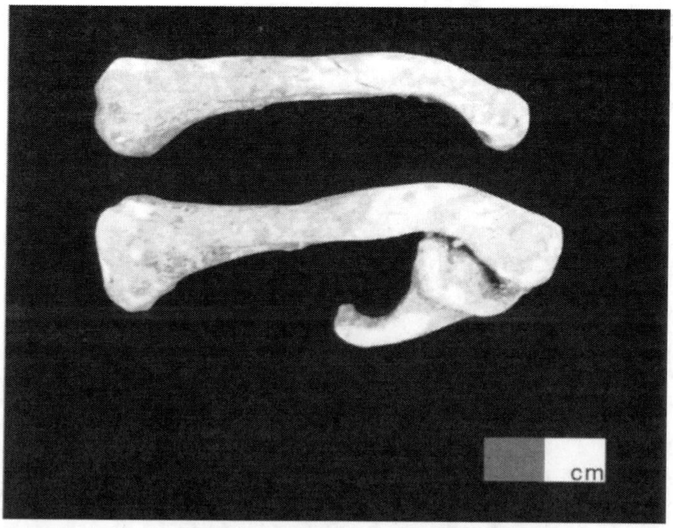

Figure 2. Abnormal proximal phalanges left middle finger.

- The hand (see Figure 2-3 (7): He is the first prehistoric skeleton found to have an abnormal left middle finger with a brachymesophalangia type 2A. The left proximal and middle phalanges of his middle finger were volarly and radially curved. Taking into consideration his hand and upper limb deformities, it is unlikely that he had full function of the upper limb.
- The spine: His vertebral column was laterally curved indicating that he also had idiopathic scoliosis. His lower lumbar vertebrae had significantly narrowed invertebrae disc spaces and osteophytes. This would have caused him to walk with a limp (see Figure 1).

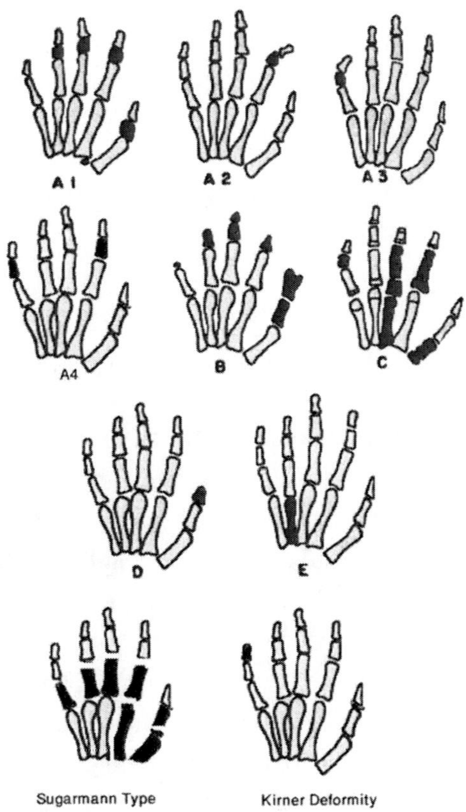

Figure 3. Main types of isolated brachydactyly.

- The lower limb: The left lower limb was noted to be markedly shorter than the right (see Figure 1) and together with the scoliosis; it is highly probable that this exaggerated the limp due to scoliosis, giving him a very abnormal gait.

DISCUSSION

The Perak Man is estimated to have died at the age of 40-45 years, which is twice the life expectancy of his time. The current knowledge of prehistoric lifespan suggests that the average lifespan of his community was 20-30 years. The way the Perak Man's body was buried indicated that he was an important person in the tribe. He was buried with both legs folded up to the chest while both hands were holding some pieces of meat. There were 2,878 riverine food shells, several types of animal flesh and 10 stone tools weighing 1.261 kg placed around him, scattered all over the burial site. This was probably an effort to ensure an abundant afterlife. This indicated that great effort was taken by his community to bury him with honour (8).

Persons with disabilities living with significant limitations in functioning often experience exclusion from full participation in their communities (4). Factors such as inaccessible physical environment, lack of relevant assistive technology and rehabilitative devices and the negative attitudes of people limit functions and create disability (9). The Perak Man with multiple disabilities, was probably unable to hunt effectively, yet he was given a more suitable role to play and was able to lead the long life of a respected person, being buried with the full honours of his time.

The community may have insulated him from death resulting from accidents or injuries, whereas others went out on the more risky job of hunting to survive. Due to the care and respect given to him by the community, he survived to a comparatively old age. He would have gained knowledge and experience in survival, planning, hunting methods, healing and related aspects of prehistoric life. He possibly took the role of a Shaman. He may have been a person who did not incorporate disability into his identity, thus taking on the special role he had in his community. Murugami (2) described situations where persons with disability have ascribed themselves as able-bodied, deeming the "biological" self as unimportant as long as they are capable of engaging in life roles as much as the persons without disabilities, in some instances doing more than their counterparts (2).

From the community perspective, protecting a member of society, who has disabilities, and giving him a more suitable role to play, including him in community life, allowed him to become more valuable to society, the longer he survived (10).

The Perak Man may have experienced and benefited from a form of community based rehabilitation (CBR). The modern world CBR was initiated by the World Health Organization (WHO) in 1978 to promote access to rehabilitation services in low and middle income countries (11). It is also seen as a strategy that helps address the ugly forms of discrimination existing in the community. The strategy focuses on enhancing the quality of life of PWDs and their families, to meet their basic needs and ensuring inclusion and participation their own development and community development (5).

When we consider current society, persons of different ability may also have heightened abilities compared to others in the remaining functions available to them. It is known that the blind hear more acutely. Even temporary blocking of one sense heightens other senses (12). It has been reported that some persons with disabilities have similar school potentials, mental functioning and educational aspirations as their non-disabled peers (2). It is possible in this age that these often more acute abilities may be made use of by society as a whole, especially where technology may enhance such opportunities.

CONCLUSION

The discovery of Perak Man and his mortuary goods has yielded extraordinary evidence of his physical condition as well as of prehistoric ways of life. The Perak Man is an example of how an ancient civilization was able to adapt roles so that a person with disabilities could use qualities available to be included in and contribute to society and to lead a long and respected life. Something that present society with all its sophistication could research, and derive benefit from, for the truly "differently" abled and society as a whole.

ACKNOWLEDGMENTS

Much of this information was found in the Lenggong Archaeological Museum. Special thanks to Emeritus Professor Datin Paduka Dr. Siti Zuraina Abdul Majid for her assistance in providing detailed information of the Perak Man in interviews and by making her research available to us. There is no potential conflict of interest reported by the authors.

REFERENCES

[1] Centers for Disease Control and Prevention. United States of America: CDC Info. URL: https://www.cdc.gov/ncbddd/disabilityandhealth/disability-barriers.html

[2] Murugami MW. Disability and identity. Disabil Stud Q 2009;29(4).

[3] Overcoming obstacles to the integration of disabled people. Disability as a human rights issue, 1995. URL: http://www.daa.org.uk/uploads/pdf/Overcoming%20Obstacles.pdf.

[4] Krahn GL, Walker DK, Correa-De-Araujo R. Persons with disabilities as an unrecognized health disparity population. Am J Public Health 2015;105(S2):S198-S206.

[5] Janardhana N, Muralidhar D, Naidu DM, Raghevendra G. Discrimination against differently abled children among rural communities in India: Need for action. J Nat Sci Biol Med 2015;6(1):7–11.

[6] Majid Z, Saidin MM, Chia SMS, Hasan Z. Artifacts from the Gua Gunung Runtuh excavations. In: Zuraina M, ed. The excavation of Gua Gunung Runtuh and the discovery of Perak man in Malaysia. Kuala Lumpur: Department of Museums and Antiquity, 1994:149-69.

[7] Temtamy SA, Aglan MS. Brachydactyly. Orphanet J Rare Dis 2008;3:15:3.

[8] Chia SMS, Majid Z. The conservation and preservation of Perak Man from Gua Gunung Runtuh site in Lenggong, Perak, Malaysia. Paper presented at: The International symposium on the conservation and Preservation of Java Man Site (Indonesia) and Peking Man Site (China), 2002 April 15-20, Solo, Indonesia.

[9] World Health Organization. International classification of functioning, disability and health. Geneva: World Health Organization, 2001.

[10] Archeological heritage of the Lenggong Valley. Volume 1. Nomination dossier for inscription on the UNESCO World Heritage List. Kuala Lumpur, Malaysia: Department of National Heritage. Ministry of Information, Communication and Culture, 2014.

[11] World Health Organization. WHO Library Cataloguing-in-publication data. Community based rehabilitation: CBR guidelines. Geneva: World Health Organization, 2010.

[12] Nilsson ME, Schenkman BN. Blind people are more sensitive than sighted people to binaural sound-location cues, particularly inter-aural level differences. Hear Res 2016;332:223–32.

In: Disability: International Aspects
Editors: Ariel Tenenbaum et al.
ISBN: 978-1-53617-886-9

Chapter 3

QUALITY OF LIFE OF FAMILIAL CAREGIVERS OF PEOPLE WITH DISABILITIES IN RURAL TAMIL NADU, INDIA

Nancy A Gnanaselvam**, MD,
Gifta P Manohari, MSW, MPhil
and Vinod Joseph Abraham, MD, MPH
Department of Community Health, St John's Medical College,
Bangalore and Department of Community Health,
Christian Medical College, Vellore, India

ABSTRACT

Caring for a family member with disability could be demanding on the life of a caregiver. Caregiver's quality of life might be adversely affected due to care giving process. This study aims to assess the quality of life of primary caregivers of people with disabilities in a rural block of Tamil

---

* Corresponding Author: Nancy Angeline Gnanaselvam, MD, Lecturer, Department of Community Health, St John's Medical College, Sarjapura Road, Bangalore, India.
E-mail: nancyangeline87@gmail.com.

Nadu, India. A total of 300 familial primary caregivers of persons with disabilities were interviewed for the study. Quality of life was assessed using the WHO QOL-BREF. Among the persons with disability, WHO Disability Assessment Schedule 2.0 was administered to assess the severity of disability. Logistic regression analysis was performed to assess the predictors of physical, psychological, social and environmental domains of quality of life of caregivers. Most caregivers were females (76%) and aged 59 years or less (70%). Mean score of physical domain (41.63) was the lowest among the domains of quality of life among the caregivers. Of the subjects, 25.7% rated their quality of life to be poor. Caregiver being female, elderly, parent or child, belonging to poor socio-economic status and presence of severe disability in the person with disability were significantly associated with poor scores in domains of quality of life. This study establishes the relationship of caregiver characteristics such as age, gender, socio-economic status, relation with the person with disability and severity of disability with the quality of life of familial caregivers of persons with disability. Caregiver support groups are vital among non formal familial caregivers for improvement for quality of life.

INTRODUCTION

Disability impacts social, economic and psychological aspects of a person's life. Societies push a person with disability to take up the role of minority status. Their social identity is defaced and this affects the individual's and family's economic status as well. Significant reduction of social contacts of a person with disability, reduced involvements in community activities and reduction in number of roles played by person can be observed as effects of disability on an individual (1). Disability not only impacts the lives of persons with disabilities but also their families, through acquisition, social, emotional and behavioural impacts. Acute illness in the family can bring the family together and improve the security levels, but chronic illness and disability in particular can be emotionally draining on the families (2). Families could take the place of institutions in taking care of a person with disability since care giving forms the core of family dynamics. Each one in the family cares for another in a unique way. The primary caregiver is defined by one who forms the patient's informal support system, takes care and responsibility of the patient and spends most of his or her time with the patient with or without any economical rewards (3).

Caregivers are viewed as an effortless alternative to meet unmet health care. However, care giving is an emotionally costly effort for caregivers (4). They can face multiple challenges due to the process of care giving. Their health can worsen due to stress, anxiety and depression. Responsibilities associated with care giving can create inconvenience in the employment conditions of a caregiver. This will have a significant impact on the economic status of the families.

In developing countries, this burden is multiplied due to inadequate health services. Poor social and employment support, illness and disturbed family life affects quality of life of caregivers negatively (5). These factors can instigate care giving burden, stress, depression and poor coping strategies among the caregivers (6). In India, approximately 90% of care is provided by family caregivers (7). The concept of trained caregivers is so far not well-known. As a result, most of the care giving is provided by untrained family members. Owing to the patriarchal society, females in the families often tend to be the caregiver (8). Most familial caregivers in India do not consider care giving as troublesome as it is a part of the family responsibility. Consequently resilience of Indian caregivers could be higher as compared to caregivers from other cultures (9). In this context, it is important to study the quality of life caregivers of persons with disability and understand the factors associated with poor quality of life.

We aimed to assess the quality of life of familial caregivers of people with disabilities in Kaniyambadi, a rural block in Tamil Nadu, India in this study. We also examined the association between quality of life of familial caregivers and characteristics of disability and socio-demographic variables

OUR STUDY

Ethical approval for the study was obtained from the Institutional Review Board, Christian Medical College, Vellore, India. All patients were provided with subject information sheet and obtained written informed consent. Consent to publish the results of the study in research journal without disclosing personal information was obtained from each subject of the study.

Participants

"Primary caregiver" in our study refers to a person who provides primary and regular care and support to a person with disability in the family. Primary caregivers aged above 18 years, related to and living with the person with disability and providing regular care and support to the person with disability were included in our study.

Study design and sampling methods

This is a community based cross sectional study done among primary caregivers of people with disabilities in Kaniyambadi– a rural block in Tamil Nadu, India. The Department of Community Health, Christian Medical College, Vellore serves this rural area and it maintains a registry of people with disabilities who are permanent residents of the block. This registry is a part of the Health Information System of the Department and is updated on a regular basis. Confirmation of diagnosis of a person with disability is done by the Community Occupational therapist and the Community Health Workers using the International Classification of Functioning, disability and health (ICF). From the registry, a complete list of adults with disability aged 18 and above residing in the block was prepared and through simple random sampling method 300 adults with disability were sampled. For our study 300 familial primary caregivers of these adults with disability were interviewed.

Instruments

The instruments used in the study were socio-demographic questionnaire, specifically developed for the study and two validated questionnaires which are described below. The socio-demographic variables studied were, age and sex of the primary caregiver, socio-economic status, type of relation to the person with disability and duration of care giving. Modified Kuppusamy socio-economic status was used to classify the socio-economic status of the study population.

World Health Organization Quality of Life Scale – BRIEF Version (WHO QOL-BREF)

The WHO QOL-BREF is a 26-item self-administered questionnaire. This questionnaire is derived from the WHO QOL-100. Each question assesses aspects of quality of life in the past 2 weeks on a 5-point scale. The first two questions measure overall quality of life and general health. There are 24 items of satisfaction with 7 items for physical health, 6 items for psychological health, 3 items for social relationships and 8 items for environmental health. Each item is rated on a 5 point likert scale. The four domain structure in WHO QOL-BREF is physical health, psychological health, social relationships and environmental factors. It is cross-culturally comparable and has sound psychometric properties (10, 11).

World Health Organization Disability Assessment Schedule (WHO DAS) 2.0

WHO DAS 2.0 is a generic assessment instrument for health and disability. It can be used across all diseases including mental diseases. It is simple to administer in both clinical and community settings. It covers 6 domains of functioning- cognition (understanding and communication), mobility (ability to move and get around), self-care (ability to attend to personal hygiene, dressing and eating, and to live alone), getting along (ability to interact with other people), life activities (ability to carry out responsibilities) and participation (ability to engage in community, civil and recreational activities) (12–14).

Statistical analysis

Statistical analysis was performed using SPSS Version 16.0. The socio demographic variables and individual questions in WHO QOL-BREF were expressed as number, percentage, mean value and standard deviation. The mean values with standard deviation of the four domains of quality of life were calculated. Chi-square test was performed to test whether there was a significant difference between the expected and observed frequencies among categorical variables. P-values of less than 0.05 were considered statistically significant. The four domains of quality of life in the WHO QOL-BREF were considered as dependent variables. To adjust for the effects of confounding variables, we added possible confounding variables which were observed to be significant in the chi square test to the regression models for each domains of quality of life and evaluated the adjusted odds ratio with 95% confidence interval. To assess for interaction between the effects of the independent variables on the quality of life of caregiver, two way ANOVA was done.

FINDINGS

Of the 300 primary caregivers of persons with disabilities interviewed, 76% were females. In our study a person aged 60 years and above was classified as elderly. A WHO DAS 2.0 score of = 45.21(45.21 was the mean score in our study) in a person with disability was termed as severe disability in our study. Baseline characteristics are described in Table 1.

Domain wise quality of life scores were calculated (see Table 2). Lowest mean score was observed for physical health (41.63). Among the subjects, 25.7% self reported quality of life to be poor and 1.7% reported very poor quality of life. Average quality of life was reported by 17% of the subjects. Dissatisfaction towards health status was reported by 26.7% of study subjects. Average satisfaction towards health status was reported by 11% of the study subjects.

Table 1. Baseline characteristics of primary caregivers

Variables		Frequency (percentage)
Gender	Male	73 (24%)
	female	227 (76%)
Age	≤59	210(70%)
	≥60	90(30%)
Relation to the person with disability	Parent or child	112 (37.30%)
	spouse	74(24.66%)
	others	114(38%)
Type of disability among persons with disability	physical	203(67.7%)
	mental	39(13%)
	physical and mental	58(19.3%)
Duration of care giving	Mean 19.66 years	SD 1.23 years
Socio-economic status	lower	36(12.0%)
	upper lower	175(58.3%)
	lower-middle	77(25.7%)
	upper-middle	12(4.0%)

Table 2. Domain wise quality of life scores for the primary caregivers of people with disabilities

Domains	Mean	Median	Standard deviation	Minimum	Maximum
Physical	41.63	42.85	6.11	17.86	60.71
Psychological	58.59	62.50	9.51	29.17	75.00
Social	65.94	75.00	14.31	16.67	100.00
Environmental	66.27	70.31	11.19	31.25	93.75

Regression analysis was performed to assess the predictors of the four domains of quality of life (see Table 3). A two way ANOVA was performed to understand the interaction between the independent variables namely, sex of the primary caregiver, caregiver being elderly, caregiver being a parent or child, poor socio-economic status and severe disability on the quality of life (see Table 4). Significant interaction was observed between the effects of parent or child being a caregiver, poor socio-economic status and severity of disability (p value 0.04) and the effects of primary caregiver being elderly, poor socio-economic status and severity of disability (p value 0.04).

Table 3. Predictors of domains of quality of life of primary care givers of people with disabilities

Domains	Variable	Unadjusted odds ratio (95% CI)	Adjusted odds ratio (95% CI)	P value
Physical	Female caregiver	0.92 (0.54-1.56)	1.07 (0.60-1.92)	0.79
	Elderly caregiver	1.96 (1.19-3.23)	1.76 (1.00-3.08)	0.05
	Caregiver being a parent or child	1.74 (1.08 – 2.79)	1.35 (0.8- 2.28)	0.26
	Poor socio-economic status	1.82 (1.09 – 3.04)	1.61 (0.94-2.76)	0.81
	Severe disability	2.13 (1.34 – 3.39)	2.04 (1.25-3.31)	0.004
Psychological	Female caregiver	1.73 (1.0 – 2.98)	2.24 (1.19-4.23)	0.01
	Elderly caregiver	3.22 (1.92 – 5.4)	3.9 (2.15-7.07)	<0.001
	Caregiver being a parent or child	2.21 (1.39 – 3.53)	1.8 (1.07-3.02)	0.03
	Poor socio-economic status	2.69 (1.58 – 4.57)	2.07 (1.64-3.7)	0.01
	Severe disability in the person with disability	3.0 (1.88 – 4.83)	2.78 (1.42-5.46)	0.003
Social	Female caregiver	3.2 (1.66 – 6.16)	4.317 (2.0-9.29)	<0.001
	Elderly caregiver	2.44 (1.47 – 4.06)	3.29 (1.77-6.13)	<0.001
	Caregiver being a parent or child	1.94 (1.19 – 3.16)	1.50 (0.86 – 2.63)	0.15
	Poor socio-economic status	4.14 (2.2 – 7.79)	2.95 (1.49-5.81)	0.002
	Severe disability in the person with disability	3.54 (2.15 – 5.81)	1.26 (0.61- 2.59)	0.53
Environmental	Female caregiver	2.18 (1.26- 3.76)	2.71 (1.43-5.13)	0.002
	Elderly caregiver	2.49 (1.49 -4.16)	2.98 (1.63-5.44)	<0.001
	Caregiver being a parent or child	2.08 (1.31-3.29)	1.64 (0.98- 2.77)	0.06
	Poor socio-economic status	2.99 (1.77-5.04)	2.31 (1.31-4.09)	0.004
	Severe disability in the person with disability	3.39 (2.11-5.46)	3.48 (2.04-5.94)	<0.001

Table 4. Interaction between variables on the quality of life of primary caregiver

Variables	F	P value
Female caregiver Parent or child caregiver Elderly caregiver	0.05	0.82
Female caregiver Parent of child caregiver Poor socio-economic status	0.26	0.60
Female caregiver Parent of child caregiver Severity of disability	0.90	0.34
Female caregiver Elderly caregiver Poor socio-economic status	0.70	0.40
Female caregiver Elderly caregiver Severity of disability	1.66	0.19
Female caregiver Poor socio-economic status Severity of disability	1.41	0.23
Parent or child caregiver Elderly caregiver Poor socio-economic status	2.02	0.15
Parent or child caregiver Elderly caregiver Severity of disability	0.98	0.32
Parent or child caregiver Poor socio-economic status Severity of disability	4.17	0.04
Elderly caregiver Poor socio-economic status Severity of disability	4.35	0.04

DISCUSSION

Among the 300 familial primary caregivers in our study, 27.4% rated their quality of life as poor. Most of the primary caregivers had negative feelings often (92.4%). Caregivers experiencing burn out and strain due to care giving activities is commonly observed (15). Dissatisfaction towards health status was reported by 26.7% of study subjects. The observed dissatisfaction about their health could have risen from the additional responsibility of care giving. Mental health status of the primary caregiver, especially depression and coping skills was not assessed in our study. Further studies can be done to understand the mental health status of caregivers of persons with disabilities.

Available studies on the quality of life of caregivers reveal that caregiver's quality of life is lower as compared to the general population (16, 17). In our study we observed the mean score of physical, psychological, social and environmental domain were 41.63, 58.69, 65.94 and 66.27 respectively. In a study done among caregivers of children and adolescents with disabilities, the mean score of each domain in WHO QOL-BREF were physical 13.71 ± 2.35, mental 12.21 ± 2.55, social 12.99 ± 2.43 and environment 12.32 ± 2.3 (16). The difference in the mean scores of domains of quality of life in our study as compared to this study could be due to the difference in the profile of persons being cared for and the caregivers. In Indian families, care giving is considered as a fulfilling experience. In a country with limited institutional facilities and welfare supports, joint families, even with little or no care giving experience and training, form a major support for persons with chronic illnesses (4).

Resilience and cultural beliefs about caring for a family member could have contributed to the apparently higher quality of life scores among our study population. In our study, 26.7% of the caregivers were dissatisfied about their health. Similar to our findings, physical health and economical status of the caregiver being affected by care giving was observed by Lecovich (18). In traditional familial relationships, taking care of people with disabilities with little or no support from societies and the Government could take a toll on the health and economic status of the care giver and the family members. Care giving negatively affecting physical health of the caregiver needs to be studied further, given that the wealth of evidence on caregiver health focuses on the burden and stress and not on physical health of caregivers (19).

In our study, caregiver characteristics such as female gender, being elderly, type of relation to the caregiver, disability characteristics such as severity and poor socio-economic status were found to be significantly associated with quality of life of primary caregivers in the regression analysis. Similar results were observed in a study done by Lin et al. among caregivers of children and adolescents with intellectual disability, where income, health status, tension and support from family were observed to correlate with all the domains of quality of life of caregivers (16). In a study done among caregivers of schizophrenics by Caqueo-Urizar et al. employment status of the caregiver and in turn economic status of the household were affected due to care giving and this adversely affected the quality of life of caregivers (20). Apart from the loss of income due to a person in the family suffering from disability, family caregivers, due to the care giving responsibilities, often forfeit their occupation. This could lead to poor socio-economic status in the family (21).

In line with our study, Morley et al. in their study among caregivers of Parkinson's disease observed that, female gender of the caregiver and caregiver being an elderly were observed to be at risk for poor quality of life (22). Although available studies on gender and care giving state that female caregivers are more prone for care giving burden and stress (23–27). The true nature and extent of this phenomenon needs to be studied further, since universally, more females take up care giving roles as compared to males and the coping strategies of females are different from males (28). Cormec et al. observed that coping skills were observed to be better among caregivers who took care of their loved ones (29).

In Indian families, good relationship with parents and children is fostered throughout life. Children consider it their fortune and responsibility to take care of their parents, since parents have loved them and taken care of them when they were young. However, in our study caregiver being a parent or child to the person with disability was significantly associated with poor quality of life in the caregiver (30). This could be attributed to the changing family dynamics in urbanizing India, where nuclear families are becoming the norm. In our study severity of disability is associated with quality of life. In line with our study, Ertekin et al. observed that higher levels of disability among multiple sclerosis patients were found to be associated with poor quality of life of their caregivers (31). Chou et al. and Leung et al. in their studies have shown that the quality of life of caregivers of persons with intellectual disabilities is associated with the severity of disability (32, 33). Presence of more impairments and severe disability in the person with disability can demand more attention and care from the caregiver, thereby impacting negatively the caregiver's quality of life.

Caring for a person with disability is a challenging task. It can be physically and mentally demanding for the caregivers. In our study female and elderly caregivers, poor socio-economic status in the family and severe disability in the person with disability are factors associated with poor quality of life among caregivers of persons with disability. Community based rehabilitation of persons with disability and support groups among caregivers could improve the quality of life of caregivers of people with disabilities.

Acknowledgments

This study was funded by the fluid research grants, Christian Medical College, Vellore.

References

[1] Stolov WC, Clowers MR. Psychosocial adjustments to chronic disease and disability. Handbook of severe disability: A text for rehabilitation counselors, other vocational practitioners and allied health professionals. Washington, DC: US Department Education Rehabilitation Services Administration, 1981.

[2] Aldridge J, Becker S. Children as carers: The impact of parental illness and disability on children's caring roles. J Fam Ther 1999;21(3):303–20.

[3] Dwyer W. J, Lee R. G, Jankowski TB. Reciprocity, elder satisfaction, and caregiver stress and burden: The exchange of aid in the family care giving relationship. J Marriage Fam 1994;56(1):35–43.

[4] Murthy Rs. Caregiving and caregivers: Challenges and opportunities in India. Indian J Soc Psychiatry 2016;32(1):10.

[5] Caqueo-Urizar A, Maldonado JG, Miranda-Castillo C. Quality of life in caregivers of patients with schizophrenia: A literature review. Health Qual Life Outcomes 2009;7:84.

[6] Glozman JM. Quality of life of caregivers. Neuropsychol Rev 2004;14(4):183–96.

[7] Kaplan D, Berkman B. The Oxford handbook of social work in health and aging. Second. Oxford: Oxford University Press, 2015.

[8] Bains P, Minhas AS. Profile of home-based caregivers of bedridden patients in North India. Indian J Commun Med 2011;36(2):114–9.

[9] Jagannathan A. Family caregiving in India: Importance of need-based support and intervention in acute care settings. J Postgrad Med 2014;60(4):355.

[10] WHOQOL-BREF: Introduction, administration, scoring and generic version of the assessment? Field trial version. Institutional Repository for Information Sharing 1996. URL: http://apps.who.int/iris/handle/10665/63529?mode=full&submit_simple=Show+full+item+record.

[11] World Health Organization. Measuring quality of life. WHO QOL. Geneva: Division on Mental Health and Substance Abuse, 1997. URL: http://www.who.int/mental_health/media/68.pdf.

[12] Luciano JV, Ayuso-Mateos JL, Aquado J, Fernandez A, Serrano-Clanco A, Roca M, et al. The 12 Item World Health Organization Disability Assessment Schedule II (WHO-DAS II): A nonparametric item response analysis. BMC Med Res Methodol 2010;10:45.

[13] Garin O, Ayuso-Mateos JL, Almansa J, Nieto M, Chatterji S. Validation of the "World Health Organization Disability Assessment Schedule, WHODAS-2" in patients with chronic diseases. Health Qual Life Outcomes 2010;8:51.

[14] World Health Organization. WHO Disability Assessment Schedule 2.0 WHODAS 2.0 2016. URL: http://www.who.int/classifications/icf/whodasii/en/

[15] Van den Heuvel ET, De Witte LP, Schure LM, Sanderman R, Meyboom-de Jong B. Risk factors for burn-out in caregivers of stroke patients, and possibilities for intervention. Clin Rehabil 2001;15(6):669–77.

[16] Lin, Jin-Ding, Jung, Yen, Chia-Feng, Hsu. Quality of life in caregivers of children and adolescents with intellectual disabilities: Use of WHOQOL-BREF survey. Res Dev Disabil 2009;30(6):1448–58.

[17] Wong DFK, Lam AYK, Chan SK, Chan SF. Quality of life of caregivers with relatives suffering from mental illness in Hong Kong: roles of caregiver characteristics, care giving burdens, and satisfaction with psychiatric services. Health Qual Life Outcomes 2012;10:15.

[18] Iecovich E. Caregiving burden, community services, and quality of life of primary caregivers of frail elderly persons. J Appl Gerontol 2008;27(3):309–30.

[19] Shaji KS, Reddy MS. Caregiving: A public health priority. Indian J Psychol Med 2012;34(4):303–5.

[20] Caqueo-Urízar A, Gutiérrez-Maldonado J, Miranda-Castillo C. Quality of life in caregivers of patients with schizophrenia: A literature review. Health Qual Life Outcomes 2009;7:84.

[21] Chadda RK. Caring for the family caregivers of persons with mental illness. Indian J Psychiatry 2014;56(3):221–7.

[22] Morley D, Dummett S, Peters M, Kelly L, Hewitson P, Dawson J, et al. Factors influencing quality of life in caregivers of people with Parkinson's disease and implications for clinical guidelines. Parkinson's disease. Parkinson's Disease 2012 (2012):190901. Doi:10.1155/2012/190901.

[23] Ysti MM, Strandberg T, Savikko N, Tilvis RS, Eloniemi-Sulkava U. Gender differences in dementia spousal caregiving. Int J Alzheimers Dis 2012 (2012):162960. Doi: 10.1155/2012/162960.

[24] Akpinar B, Küçükgüçlü O, Yener G. Effects of gender on burden among caregivers of Alzheimer's patients. J Nurs Scholarsh 2011;43(3):248–54.

[25] Kao H-FS, McHugh ML. The role of caregiver gender and caregiver burden in nursing home placements for elderly Taiwanese survivors of stroke. Res Nurs Health 2004;27(2):121–34.

[26] Pinquart M, Sorensen S. Gender differences in caregiver stressors, social resources, and health: An updated meta-analysis. J Gerontol B Psychol Sci Soc Sci 2005.18;61(1):33–45.

[27] Gallicchio L, Siddiqi N, Langenberg P, Baumgarten M. Gender differences in burden and depression among informal caregivers of demented elders in the community. Int J Geriatr Psychiatry 2002;17(2):154–63.

[28] Sharma N, Chakrabarti S, Grover S. Gender differences in caregiving among family - caregivers of people with mental illnesses. World J Psychiatry 2016;6(1):7–17.

[29] Cormac I, Tihanyi P. Meeting the mental and physical healthcare needs of carers. Adv Psychiatr Treat 2006;(12):162–72.

[30] Lukhmana S, Bhasin SK, Chhabra P, Bhatia MS. Family caregivers' burden: A hospital based study in 2010 among cancer patients from Delhi. Indian J Cancer 2015;52(1):146.

[31] Ertekin Ö, Özakbas S, Idiman E. Caregiver burden, quality of life and walking ability in different disability levels of multiple sclerosis. Neuro Rehabil 2014;34(2):313–21.

[32] Chou YC, Schalock RL, Tzou PY, Lin LC, Chang AL, Lee WP, et al. Quality of life of adults with intellectual disabilities who live with families in Taiwan. J Intellect Disabil Res 2007;51(11):875–83.

[33] Yuen Shan Leung C, Wai Ping Li-Tsang C. Quality of life of parents who have children with disabilities. Hong Kong J Occupat Ther 2003;13(1):19–24.

In: Disability: International Aspects
Editors: Ariel Tenenbaum et al.
ISBN: 978-1-53617-886-9

Chapter 4

INTERRELATIONSHIP BETWEEN FAMILY, POVERTY AND SOCIAL PROTECTION IN UGANDA: PERSPECTIVES OF PERSONS WITH DISABILITIES

Beatrice A Alupo*[1], *BA, MA, MSc,
Maxwell P Opoku*[2,*], *BA, MSc, MSc,
Eric Badu*[3], *BA, MSc
and Wisdom K Mprah*[3], *BA, MPhil, PhD
[1]School of Government and International Relations, Griffith University, Brisbane, Queensland, Australia
[2]Faculty of Education, University of Tasmania, Launceston, Tasmania, Australia
[3]Centre for Disability Rehabilitation, Kwame Nkrumah University of Science and Technology, Kumasi, Ghana

[*] Corresponding Author's E-mail: maxwell.opoku@utas.edu.au.

Abstract

Persons with disabilities encounter numerous barriers that prevent them from participating in society on an equal basis with others. They also have limited opportunities and choices and therefore are more likely to have lower educational achievements, poorer health outcomes, lower employment rates, and live in poorer housing conditions than their counterparts without disabilities. Discourse on the need to improve the life of persons with disabilities has not fully explored the relationship between formal and informal social protection when it comes to explaining their living conditions. This chapter explore the life experiences of persons with disabilities in the Kampala Metropolitan Area in Uganda. A qualitative study using in-depth interviews was conducted with 30 participants using a convenient sampling technique to explore participants' life experiences. As expected, participants in the study area were dissatisfied with their current state of living, but there were limited opportunities to transform the situation. This is because there were no effective safety nets to support vulnerable populations such as persons with disabilities in Uganda. More innovative policies and programs, that will strengthen traditional forms of social support systems, while providing a more comprehensive social protection for the majority of the population, is proposed.

Introduction

In every society around the world, persons with disabilities are highly over-represented among the poor (1-3). Disability deepens vulnerabilities to poverty such that persons with disabilities are likely to be denied access to services that will improve their lives (4, 5). The passage of the Convention on the Rights of Persons with Disabilities [CRPD] introduced a new era where signatory states were expected to promulgate laws aimed at maximizing the potential of persons with disabilities. This human right approach proposed inclusive development where social, political, civil and economic barriers will be overcome to ensure the full participation of persons with disabilities in communal life (6, 7). However, little has been achieved regarding improvements in the living standards of persons with disabilities, as many tend to rely on the benevolence of society for survival (8, 9).

Begging has been branded as a demeaning act which affects the individual's self-worth and dignity (8, 10). Both international and national legal frameworks make provision for introduction of deliberate policies to enhance the dignity of persons with disabilities to enable them to have means of livelihood without relying on others or engaging in acts such as begging to survive. In Uganda, the 1995 constitution is clear and upholds the need to safeguard the rights of persons with disabilities through the promulgation of laws by Parliament. However, the interaction between beliefs, social expectations and even poverty affects the support society is expected to give to persons with disabilities (11, 12). For instance, in most societies in Uganda, there is a stigma associated with a disability which results in families uninterested in supporting their members living with disabilities (12, 13). This to some extent explains the poor performance and low participation of persons with disabilities in areas that would lift them out of poverty.

Persons with disabilities are unable to participate equally in productive social activities as their peers (9, 11). This is evident in their low participation in education, employment, healthcare, social life and asset ownership as any other persons in the society (13-15). Due to poor infrastructure and lack of teaching and learning materials in schools in Uganda, there is little chance for children with disabilities to have access to education (12, 15). In a sense, disability limits children from schooling more than other factors such as the area of residence (rural or urban), gender and economic status. The inability of persons with disabilities to participate in education pervades other areas of their lives which deepen their vulnerability to poverty. Without requisite education qualification, the ability of persons with disabilities to compete for the limited job opportunities would be minimal (2, 11, 16). The inability of persons with disabilities to engage in economic activities become a burden on society, family and dependents. It is unsurprising that household with a person with disability as head is reportedly 38% poorer than households headed by a person without a disability (17). This reinforces the link between disability and the long run vicious cycle of poverty among persons with disabilities and their families.

The lack of opportunities and avenue for persons with disabilities to overcome or break social barriers make them susceptible in the society. Understandably, most of them move out of home or their community in search of their daily bread (8, 10, 16). Thus, this study aims to involve persons with disabilities who are on the streets in Uganda to share their experiences and activities for daily living. For the purpose of this study, disability is defined as the barriers in the society which affect the social, political and economic participation of individuals living with impairments (3, 18). In this article, we argued that the absence of family support and weak state sponsored social protection make life unbearable for the majority of persons with disabilities. Drawing upon a qualitative research, this paper explored the life experiences of persons with disabilities living on the streets in Uganda. The study adopted a qualitative data collection method, using in-depth interviews. The design provided an opportunity to explore participants' life experiences and provided insightful evidence of individual life experiences of persons with disabilities who were mainly living on the streets to make a living.

Social protection in Uganda

As in many African societies, indigenous populations in Uganda had ways of supporting themselves long before the advent of formal social protection programs (19). The traditional Ugandan society is communal and closely knitted as the extended family was extensive, and everyone was linked up with all the other members, including the living and dead, in a complex web of social and spiritual relationships (20-22). Responsibility was collective and based on moral reciprocity, so there was a shared responsibility and strong mutual support. Hence, individuals considered themselves integral in the larger community, and any act committed by a member of the extended family or any misfortune that befell a member was perceived collective, and every member participated in remedying the situation (19, 23, 24). This implies that conformity was highly valued, and thus, it was an obligation for every member to uphold the values of the community, because any deviant behaviour could affect the stability of the whole community.

Despite the existence of communalism and each other's keeper, disability was not tolerated in traditional African society. The perception was that everyone has to play their part to keep the society and practices intact. When a male child is born, during naming ceremony, the machete was placed on them as a sign of hard work and initiation into the world work. However, having a disability was seen as a burden because the individual was deemed unfit to make a substantial contribution to the communal practices (1, 5, 9, 10). In most societies in Uganda, there is an outright rejection of individuals who do not possess the "body form" which is seen as normal (11, 12). For instance, Stone-MacDonald and Butera (25) mentioned that children with disabilities were not accepted in communities because they are seen as sub-humans who would be unproductive. Hence, the common practices were to guide against having a child with a disability who might not be able to support the community – though they were supported and provided food for their daily living.

However, modernization and migration in Uganda have destabilised the traditional communal system which has made the traditional social protection system ineffective (19, 24). The movement of people from their traditional societies signified their departure from communalism that existed in their ancestral homes (22). These events led to the introduction of money as the only medium of exchange, caused indigenous populations to lose their right to manage their affairs and migration to urban areas for greener pastures. The consequences were the disintegration of the traditional extended family system, and values, such as reciprocity and social cohesion became irrelevant. The indigenous social security system was, therefore, adversely affected due to frequent movement of people, thus, denying families the chance to live together in one community and support one another (24). Consequently, vulnerable groups no more received the support they got from the extended family.

As the traditional social security eroded and poverty in Uganda worsened, the need to protect vulnerable groups became imperative. The Government of Uganda, therefore, introduced formal social protection programs to cushion the effects of poverty on vulnerable populations (6, 23, 24). One of such programs is the Expanding Social Protection (ESP) program, which was launched in 2010 (19, 26, 27). The goal of the ESP program is to protect "vulnerable groups (that is the elderly, people with disabilities and the poorest of the poor) from deprivation and livelihood risks by initiating policies and promoting development programs and projects that protect the rights of these vulnerable groups (26). The diverse nature of the program has increased the resilience of beneficiaries as they can invest in economic activities such as commercial farming, shops, restaurants and even expanding workshops. Although formal social protection programmes, such as the ESP have chalked some successes, they have been criticized for being ineffective in alleviating poverty among vulnerable populations (22). Although the purpose of the study was not to review the impact of social protection programs on persons with disabilities, the study will provide some understanding into the effectiveness of social protection programs on groups that have unique needs and whose needs may be invisible, for example, persons with disabilities.

OUR STUDY

Participation was voluntary as there was no reward, but after each interview, the participant was served with lunch. In all, 36 people attended the meeting: six persons with visual impairment, 17 persons with physical impairment and 13 persons with hearing impairment. All the six persons with visual impairment agreed to participate and were recruited. Of the 17 persons with physical disabilities, 14 decided to participate while ten persons with hearing impairment, out of the 13 agreed to participate, making 30 participants. On reaching 30 participants, we decided not to continue with the recruitment when we realized that no new information was emerging (28).

All the participants were taken through informed consent process which was orally read to participants before they were recruited. The informed consent process involved informing participants about the purpose of the study, its voluntary nature, the duration and their right to withdraw at any point during the study. They were also assured of the anonymity and confidentiality of their identity. Although the informed consent was written in English, it was translated to Luganda which is the language spoken by many people in the study area and the Uganda Sign Language for participants with hearing disabilities. To ensure the privacy of the participants and to avoid disruptions, all the interviews were conducted in an office we rented.

Procedure for data collection

The study and its protocol were approved by Institute of Governance, Humanities and Social Sciences, Pan African University, Cameroon. Afterwards, we sought authorization from Uganda National Council for Science and Technology (UNCST) before the data collection. The interviews were conducted on five different occasions in June 2015 by the first and third author at City Square in Kampala. Participants were recruited through announcements made through public address system and posted a notice at the entrance of Saint Balikuddembe market which is the main market in Kampala. Additionally, a formal letter was sent to the executive of the various disability associations, informing them of the study and inviting their members to participate in the study. Also, we moved on the streets and invited persons with disabilities who were engaged in begging and selling at the market to participate in the study. On the day of data collection, those who came were educated about the study and its objectives. The major issues covered in the interview were the background characteristics of participants, sources of livelihood, family support, access to education, occupation and their views of family and state-engineered social support.

Data collection method

The instrument for data collection was semi-structured interview guide developed based on the objectives of the study and literature (1, 6, 8, 10, 29). Each participant was interviewed once for at least one hour. Although the interview guide was written in English, participants spoke in Luganda, which is the primary language spoken by most people in Uganda. The interview was conducted by first and third authors who were supported by a hired research assistant who is fluent in English and sign language. All the interviews were audio-recorded with permission from the participants. For persons with hearing disabilities, the researchers asked the questions while the interpreter translated them into Ugandan Sign Language for participants with hearing disabilities. The interpreter voiced their responses into audio-recorder.

Data management and analysis

We performed content analysis following the steps described by (30). The third author and the research assistant translated all the audio recordings orally and separately from Luganda to English onto an audio-recorder. Afterwards, they listened to the audio recordings from the two translations and differences in the translations identified and reconciled. The audio recordings were then professionally transcribed to Microsoft word. We all read the transcription several times and addressed discrepancies. Using our research questions (each research question was given a numerical code) as the framework, each researcher analysed the data separately. While reading the transcribed data, we identified and categorised codes that were relevant to the research questions using the numerical codes. We then met to discuss the categories, and similar categories were merged under themes.

FINDINGS

The majority of participants (70%) were males; over 40% of them were between 26 and 35 years while 10% were between 46 and 55 years with a mean age of 31 years. More than half (56.7%) of the participants had not formal education – only 3.3% had formal education up to tertiary level (post-secondary qualification). As expected, a significant number of the participants (43.3%) were unemployed. Those who were employed were civil servants (13.3%), artisan (20%) and traders (23%). It is important to mention that majority (74.5%) of those who said they were employed as civil servants engaged in menial jobs such as labourers and cleaners.

Table 1. Socio-demographic characteristics of participants

Variable	Frequency	Percentage (%)
Age (years)		
• 18 – 25	6	20
• 26 – 35	13	43.3
• 36 – 45	8	26.7
• 46- 55	3	10
Total	30	100
Mean age (years)	31	
Marital status		
• Married	3	10
• Single	19	63.3
• Divorced	8	26.7
Total	30	100
Level of education		
• None	17	56.7
• Primary	9	30
• Secondary	3	10
• Tertiary	1	3.3
Total	30	100
Employment		
• Artisan	6	20
• Civil Servant	4	13.3
• Trading	7	23.3
• Unemployed	13	43.3
Total	30	100

Table 1. (Continued)

Variable	Frequency	Percentage (%)
Disability type		
• Physical impaired	14	46.7
• Visual impaired	6	20
• Hearing impaired	10	33.3
Total	30	100
Number of children		
• 0	15	50
• 1-3	8	26.7
• 4-6	3	10
• 7≤	4	13.3
Total	30	100

Source: Field data, 2015

The traders were mainly in petty trading such as selling fruits, necklace, and candies, while the artisans involved in carpentry, shoemaking and craftwork. All traders and artisans do not own shops; rather they sold their wares on pavements along the roads and streets. Divorce appears to be high among the participants as eight (26.7%) out the 30 participants said, they were divorced; only 10% (3) were married. Table 1 below presents a summary of participants' socio-demographic characteristics

Isolation, rejection and abuse

Responses from participants suggested that many encountered social isolation, rejection and abuse from family members, spouses and neighbors. Most of them claimed that their families abandoned because of their impairment. Some claimed they did not even know where their families were and did not consider themselves part of their biological families. Two persons with visual disability and a person with hearing disability narrated their experiences:

> I was dumped, so I do not have a family. I do not hear from my family members because they dislike me. I have to stay on my own and

survive. No one was ready to support me, so I have to stay away from them [Visually disability 2, male].

I have no relatives now. We don't relate very much because of the disability. We lived peacefully but since I became disabled, nobody was prepared to take care of me. They used to give maximum care but now I'm not welcome in my family. They don't want to see me around, and I have driven away [Visually disability 4, male].

My family abandoned me when I had this disability. I have no family. I rely only on well-wishers for my support. None of my family members check on me to give me money or food. I take care of myself [Hearing disability 8, male].

Apart from the effects of disability on blood relations, marriages were also affected as the acquisition of disability resulted in the breakdown of few marriages, leaving the spouses who became disabled to fend for themselves, and sometimes, their children alone.

My wife ran off with my three children when it was confirmed that I wouldn't be able to see again. I don't know their whereabouts that is why you find me here under the hot sun trying to survive. That's not what I want to do, but I have to do it to survive [visual disability 5, female].

I look after myself. My wife and family have all abandoned me. I have a friend who is rich who has given me a job to wash his cars than going to beg people on the street. This is a time I need support but they are nowhere to be found but life goes on [hearing disability 2, male].

Although as adults they were supposed to be independent of their family members, having a disability, mainly acquiring it later in life, require some support for one to adapt to the changes that have taken place in one's life. The transformation individuals might have gone through, could affect their relationship with the family. Hence, without any help, the chances of people developing their potentials and becoming productive diminished.

Lack of education

The narratives below suggest that most participants did not receive a formal education because family members were unwilling to invest in their education. This was confirmed by some participants, who indicated that family members and friends thought they were unproductive and could not do anything for themselves and their communities. Therefore, it was considered a waste of resources investing in their education.

> No one wants to educate disabled, and I have affected the same reason. My family thinks I can't study and did not do much to take me to school. I'm always sad seeing people and my colleagues I grow up with go to school, but I'm here doing nothing [visual disability 2, male].
>
> I have no relevant education qualification. I have not been to school. My family thinks I'm disabled, so I can't learn, but that is not the case. I can learn as any other person. Even the schools are far, and it would have been difficult for me to attend [visual disability 6, male]

Additionally, some participants mentioned that their inability to have access to education was due to lack of financial support which led to school dropout.

> I stopped schooling at Primary 3. I lacked school fees to continue. Even in government schools, you are supposed to pay so without money I couldn't stay in school. Money was an obstacle to enable me realized my dream [Visual disability 3, male].
>
> I wished to be a lawyer one day, but this disability affected my dream. It is sad that because of money and lack of support I have to stay on the street. I know that if I had been to school, I would have been in my office [Physical disability 3, male].

It is therefore not surprising to have more than half of the participants without any formal education. Moreover, without formal education, opportunities are limited, and one is compelled to live at the mercy of benevolence as discussed by participants.

Lack of gainful employment

As the demographic characteristics of participants indicated, the majority of participants were either unemployed or employed in low paid jobs. This situation seems to be due to lack of formal education and negative attitudes towards persons with disabilities. Two participants confirmed this assertion.

> No one will employ you when he or she sees that you have not gone to school and having disability make it worse. It is about qualification first even if someone wants to consider you for a job; I have no certificate to show present for such jobs [Hearing disability 9, female].
>
> I am not working because I couldn't access education. It's difficult to get a job since those not disabled are the ones preferred by the government and other employers. We have no chance getting jobs in this country making us dependent on others [Hearing disability 1, male].

Communication barriers (for example, lack of sign language interpreters) and lack of support services such as accessible information to persons with visual disabilities at workplaces was also blamed for their inability to secure jobs.

> Communication is a significant barrier restricting our ability to work. I use sign language to communicate, and not all people understand. It was working so I cannot work anywhere. It's hard to communicate, and that is my problem [Hearing disability 1, female].
>
> I have the strength to work, but my inability to talk disqualifies me all the time. It would have been easier if I have a personal interpreter all the time, but no employer will do that in this country. That is a big issue for us, but we can't do anything at the moment [Physical disability 13, male].
>
> Offices do not have braille machines to enable us to work so even if they employ us we cannot function to our ability due to some of these restrictions. If these things are available, it would have motivated most of us to go to school [Visual disability 6, male].

Most participants mentioned that the physical environment restricts their ability to move freely which deny them the opportunity to participate in social and economic activities. Although laws have been made to make all buildings accessible, they were not being enforced

> I am glad you have asked me that question. I hear that it is in the constitution to build structures to accommodate persons with disabilities. However, our government has not taken up this issue. Private companies put up structures that do not accommodate the need of persons with disabilities making it difficult for us to go to them for jobs [Visual disability 1, female].

Due to limited opportunities, begging on the street to make a living has become the option for some participants. Without family support and funds to start-up their businesses, some participants said that they had to stay on the streets and beg passer-by to survive on a daily basis. Three participants explained as follows:

> I stay alone and cater for myself without any support from my family members. I beg and people who love and care give me money. I don't do anything productive, and I hope to find something doing one day [Physical disability 2, female].
>
> I have nothing doing because of my disability. I just come here in the traffic jam and beg for money from those who are kind enough to help me. No one from the family assists me and I have to survive daily. I look after myself [Physical disability 1, male].
>
> I can't do anything than to beg from people. Persons with disability have a right of being given or helped by those who are well off. We are like a test to those who are wealthy, and God expects them to assist us with money and our needs [visual disability 3, male].

Although begging is considered 'unproductive', it was justified as the only means of survival for some participants.

Inadequate government support

There were differing opinions regarding assistance being provided by the governments. While some participants claimed they had received some support from the government, although it was inadequate to engage in anything profitable with it, others said they had not received any assistance from the government.

> I do get some money, but it is not much. The problem is that the money occasionally comes, so it's hard for me to plan using it for the intended purpose. I just use to cover hospital bills and settle people I have borrowed money from [Visual disability 3, male].
>
> The government is trying to do something, but I have seen that the support comes when we make noise. The money is so little, and I wish I could have much money to trade. I only get something small [Physical disability 4, male].

However, some participants said they had never received any support from the government. Several participants also discussed that they are unable to access political support due to lack of information on where, when and how they could benefit from such governmental initiatives. The following quotations summarise experiences of participants:

> The government doesn't help us, but we are also citizens whose needs should be considered. They should assist us to move out from the streets. They have not been helping us. We need help, but it seems like no one is ready to help us move out of the street. I wish I could leave here and work somewhere [Hearing disability 7, male].
>
> I have never got any help from the government. Mainly the only help is from NGOs. I do hear of other people who at times get something from the government, but I don't know where to go or who to talk to get such assistance [Visual disability 1, female].
>
> I'm told the government give money to disabled persons, but I don't know how to apply. There is no need to continue begging if I'm able to access the funds. If you don't know anyone in government, there is no way you would get that information. I don't know and none of my friends who beg also don't know [Physical disability 9, male].

The assertions by participants on their inability to have access to government support might suggest that guidelines have not been put in place or even if there is, they seemed not to be followed when it comes to disbursement of funds. Also, it is fair to allude that the cash seemed not to reach the core poor on the streets who are begging to survive.

DISCUSSION

Family play a crucial role in helping persons with disabilities to develop a stable future which can significantly have an influence on their lives (31). Supportive and responsive families could encourage and motivate them to acquire life skills for independent living (32). It is, therefore, essential that persons with disabilities be given equal attention in terms love, access to education, work, and socialisation to enable them to become productive citizens of their communities. However, the results of the study revealed that persons with disabilities in the study area lacked family support. That is, the failure of family members to accept them as human and part of the family; had adverse consequences on their overall development (support services and access to necessities of life such as education), and more especially, their exclusion from society (15-17). For example, the study found that the failure of family members to support their members with disabilities to acquire formal education made it impossible for them to gain the knowledge and skills required on the labour market. Acquiring formal education would have increased their social participation, and make them competitive in the job market or even enable some have access to jobs (2, 8, 16). This finding is consistent with previous studies which found that if families reject persons with disabilities, they are likely to grow up into adults with low self–esteem and status in societies (10, 32).

As explained previously, in Uganda, the extended family acts as security and protects its members. Being abandoned by family members, or not having relatives, as claimed by participants, is inconsistent with the traditional communal setup. Perhaps, the attitude of family members towards their members with disabilities may have been influenced by deep-rooted misconceptions about disability (5, 12). Although under the traditional Uganda communal system, everyone is part of the extended family system and support for the needy is highly valued, persons with disabilities may not qualify for such support. In many African societies, including Uganda, disability is associated with evil and highly stigmatised (11, 12, 25). Apparently, families with children with disabilities may be taunted and face rejection from their neighbours. It is, therefore, a common practice for parents to hide, abandon or even kill children born with defects, such as physical impairment (33-36). The stigma attached to disability and the fact that most persons with disabilities are often considered unproductive might be major motivations for parents not to support the education of participants. These findings are somewhat in agreement with previous studies which identified shame and stigma as leading causes of rejection of children with disabilities by their family, compelling such individuals to resort to street begging (5, 8, 0).

The breakdown of the extended family system, around which the traditional or communal social protection in Uganda operate, is another possible reason for family members' attitude towards their relatives with disabilities. The traditional social security in Uganda was based on collective responsibility, and vulnerable groups were taken care of by members of the extended family (19, 24). However, social, economic and political events in Uganda, such as, the introduction of western education, wars, and the use of money as the only means of exchange, have eroded the traditional communal system, leaving vulnerable groups, who were hitherto supported by family members, to fend for themselves (24, 37). This was exactly the case in this study as participants indicated that their needs were not met by their families which had forced them to rely on themselves and discover means of survival. The family is the first agent of socialisation who have to support persons with disabilities to discover their innate potential and live independently (31, 32). As reported in this study, the family had failed to play their role which negatively impacted on the life of participants.

The growing reliance of persons with disabilities on the benevolence of society was found in this study. Coupled with limited access to education and isolation, most participants were on the streets in search of their livelihoods. Consequently, without effective policies to cater for the needs of persons with disabilities, most of them would not be able to start any productive activity. This would give them no choice than to beg to make a living – a situation evident in this study as participants who were unable to start a trade engaged in begging to survive. This practice seems to be widespread in other African countries such as Ghana (8), Kenya (16) and Nigeria (10) where begging has become an avenue for persons with disabilities to have their daily bread. Begging is derisive, and even persons with disabilities who engage in this act are aware of its devastating consequences on their self-esteem and dignity as equal members of the society. Understandably, they had no skills to apply for jobs and adaptations that could have been made to enable them to be part of the workforce are usually unavailable (11, 15, 16). The restrictive nature of physical environment as found by this study, is pervasive in several countries where public places such as schools, hospitals and major offices have been built without considerations given to the needs of persons with disabilities (2, 14, 38). This trend does not seem to be ending, as the government who is supposed to lead the fight for equal access had made little or no attempt to reform society to facilitate efforts towards inclusivity.

The intolerance of disability in some societies was re-echoed by participants of this study who claimed that despite their qualifications, they were discriminated against during job search. According to them, their disability was used as a basis for their disqualification. This could be attributed to the extent of acceptance and deep-seated perceptions society have about individuals living with disabilities (11, 15, 39). Thence, it will be fair to infer that society has consciously or unconsciously erected barriers against persons with disabilities in Uganda (6). Some participants whose marriage collapsed on the onset of their disabilities further reinforced this assertion. Admittedly, on this score, disability may have been linked to incapacity – making it difficult for them to live independently or engaged in productive economic activities (5, 10, 16). Given this unfair social order, participants turned to the streets in search of their livelihoods. In such a society, it would be fair for the government to support persons with disabilities whose impairments were used as a basis to measure their competencies.

The poor living conditions and limited opportunities have fueled the need for the institutionalised robust social protection that would cushion persons with disabilities in Uganda (9, 37, 40). However, as found by the study, the support was not forthcoming as most participants reported they had not received such support. It is important to acknowledge the fact that there was an admission of its existence but participants said they could not get access. This seems to suggest that there is an intention on the part of the Ugandan government to support persons with disabilities; however, they had not been able to reach their target (6). This could be because of the improper planning which might have resulted in the policy not trickling down to the ordinary people who had to rely on the benevolence of society to survive (41). The initiative of the state has been branded as tokenistic as it would not have any significant impact on the lives of persons with disabilities (6).

Limitations of the study

The study was limited to persons with disabilities in Kampala Metropolitan area. Hence, views expressed might not be a total representation of the situation of persons with disabilities in all over Uganda. Also, due to the small sample size, the researchers did not intend to generalise the findings. Although the study has provided insight into the living conditions of persons with disabilities in Kampala Metropolitan Area, it is important that other studies be conducted in other parts of the country to ascertain their living conditions as well.

CONCLUSION

The study documented the life experiences of persons with disabilities living in Uganda. Undoubtedly, social protection improves access to social services such as education and health, and promotes the welfare and consumptions of the beneficiaries (6). As expected, the findings of the study revealed that most persons with disabilities in the study area had to endure much hardship to make a living because of lack of support from family members and society. The results of the study have established that the breakdown of traditional and formal social protection have negated impact on the lives of persons with disabilities. With the collapse of the traditional support system and ineffective formal social protection programs, vulnerable groups in Uganda, such as persons with disabilities have been affected by current austere economic conditions and so concrete measures are needed to cushion the effects of poverty on vulnerable groups.

Efforts should be made to address the challenges hindering the efficient operation of the formal social protection programs to increase their effectiveness on poor populations in Uganda. For example, corruption and bureaucracies that make it difficult for beneficiaries to receive cash transfers should be eliminated by encouraging grassroots participation (6, 29). The government through the Uganda Bureau of Statistics should put mechanisms in place to properly target deserving beneficiaries for the ESP program (27). Also, Disability Peoples Organizations [DPOs] should push for the implementation of the numerous laws such as the Disability Act, 2006, the Equal Opportunities Commission Act 2006 and Local Government Act 1997. All these are beautiful laws, containing provisions prohibiting discrimination in all forms and have specific programmes to promote the inclusion of persons with disabilities in private and public businesses. The enforcement of these laws will go a long way in addressing the challenges persons with disabilities encounter. The capacities of the DPOs should also be strengthened through a workshop to make them more effective to advocate for the enforcement of inclusive policies and laws. While creating awareness about the equalization of opportunities for persons with disabilities among members of communities, efforts should be made to make the educational system in Uganda more generally accessible to persons with disabilities. The government should prioritize the education of persons with disabilities by providing the necessary resources, investing in the education of special educators and providing facilities. With formal education and appropriate vocational training, a person with disabilities can acquire the knowledge and skills required to be competitive in the labor market.

REFERENCES

[1] Filmer D. Disability, poverty, and schooling in developing countries: results from 14 household surveys. World Bank Econ Rev 2008;22(1):141-63.

[2] Gottlieb A, Myhill WN, Blanck P. Employment of people with disabilities. In: Stone JH, Blouin M, eds. International encyclopedia of rehabilitation. Buffalo, NY: CIRRIE, 2010:1-9.

[3] World Health Organization. World report on disability. Geneva: World Health Organization, 2011.

[4] Ingstad B, Eide A. Disability and poverty: A global challenge. World Dev 2011;33(6):995–1009.

[5] Naami A. Disability, gender, and employment relationships in Africa: The case of Ghana. Afr J Disabil 2015;4(1):1-11.

[6] Katsui H, Kumpuvuori J. Human rights based approach to disability in development in Uganda: A way to fill the gap between political and social spaces? Scand J Disabil Res 2008;10(4):227-36.

[7] Niño-Zarazúa M, Barrientos A, Hulme D, Hickey S. Social protection in Sub-Saharan Africa: Will the green shoots blossom? Manchester: Brooks World Poverty Institute, 2010.

[8] Kassah AK. Begging as work: A study of people with mobility difficulties in Accra, Ghana. Disabil Soc 2008;23(2):163-70.

[9] Mwendwa TN, Murangira A, Lang R. Mainstreaming the rights of persons with disabilities in national development frameworks. J Int Dev 2009;21(5):662-72.

[10] Edewor PA, Abimbola OH, Adekeye OA. Begging to live: The strategy of survival for people with intellectual disabilities in Nigeria. Enhancing the quality of life of people with intellectual disabilities. Netherlands: Springer, 2010:173-80.

[11] Abimanyi-Ochom J, Mannan H. Uganda's disability journey: progress and challenges: Community paper. Afr J Disabil 2014;3(1):1-6.

[12] Lwanga-Ntale C. Chronic poverty and disability in Uganda. International Conference: Staying poor: Chronic poverty and development policy, Manchester, UK, 2003.

[13] Mulumba M, Nantaba J, Brolan CE, Ruano AL, Brooker K, Hammonds R. Perceptions and experiences of access to public healthcare by people with disabilities and older people in Uganda. Int J Equity Health 2014;13(1):76.

[14] Ahumuza SE, Matovu JK, Ddamulira JB, Muhanguzi FK. Challenges in accessing sexual and reproductive health services by people with physical disabilities in Kampala, Uganda. Reprod Health 2014;11(1):59.

[15] Emong P, Eron L. Disability inclusion in higher education in Uganda: Status and strategies. Afr J Disabil 2016;5(1):1-11.

[16] Opoku MP, Kwadwo Mprah W, Dogbe JA, Moitui JN, Badu E. Access to employment in Kenya: the voices of persons with disabilities. Int J Disabil Hum Dev 2017;16(1):77-87.

[17] McClain-Nhlapo C. Including people with disabilities in actions to reduce poverty and hunger. Washington, DC: IFPRI, International Food Policy Research Institute, 2007.

[18] United Nations. Convention on the rights of persons with disabilities. New York: United Nations, 2007.

[19] Bilson A, Nyeko J, Baskott J, Rayment C. Developing social care and support services in Uganda: A situational analyses and policy recommendations. Oxford: Oxford Policy Management, 2013.

[20] Duma S. The role of social protection in the socioeconomic development of Uganda. J Soc Dev Afr 2015;10(2):5-12.

[21] Kyaddondo D, Mugisha J. Expanding social protection programme. URL: www.socialprotection.go.ug.

[22] Kyaddondo D, Mugisha J. Assessing the state of Uganda's traditional social protection systems and implications for formal social protection policy and programming. Kampala: Ministry Gender Labour Social Development, 2014.

[23] Angucia M, Katusiimeh MW. The Politics of promoting social protection in Uganda: A case of the cash transfer scheme for elderly people. Nairobi, Kenya: Partnership African Social Governance Research, 2015.

[24] Bukuluki P. The status of social security systems in Uganda: Challenges and opportunities. Kampala: Konrad Adenauer Stiftung, 2014.

[25] Stone-MacDonald A, Butera GD. Cultural beliefs and attitudes about disability in East Africa. Rev Disabil Stud 2014;8(1).

[26] Murungi I. Expanding social protection in Uganda. International Symposium: Social protection in Southern Africa. New opportunities for social development, University of Johannesburg, South Africa, 2011.

[27] Oxford Policy Management. Evaluation of the Uganda Social Assistance Grants for Empowerment (SAGE) Programme. Oxford: Baseline Report, 2013.

[28] Fusch PI, Ness LR. Are we there yet? Data saturation in qualitative research. Qual Rep 2015;20(9):1408.

[29] Hickey S. The politics of staying poor: exploring the political space for poverty reduction in Uganda. World Dev 2005;33(6):995-1009.

[30] O'Leary Z. The essential guide to doing your research project. London: Sage, 2013.

[31] Mokomane Z. Social protection as a mechanism for family protection in sub-Saharan Africa. Int J Soc Welfare 2013;22(3):248-59.

[32] McDaniel SH, Pisani AR. Family dynamics and caregiving for people with disabilities. Multiple dimensions of caregiving and disability, New York: Springer, 2012:11-28.

[33] Bleek W, Asante-Darko N. Illegal abortion in Southern Ghana: Methods, motives and consequences. Hum Organ 1986;45(4):333-43.

[34] Edewor PA, Abimbola OH, Adekeye OA. Begging to live: The strategy of survival for people with intellectual disabilities in Nigeria. Dordrecht: Springer, 2011.

[35] Baffoe M. Stigmatization, discrimination and marginalization: Gateways to oppression of persons with disabilities in Ghana, West Africa. J Educ Soc Res 2013;3(1):187-98.

[36] Kassah A. Begging as work: A study of people with mobility difficulties in Accra, Ghana. Disabil Soc 2008;23(2):163-70.

[37] Bukuluki P, Watson C. Transforming cash transfers: Beneficiary and community perceptions of the Senior Citizen Grant (SCG) in Uganda. London: Overseas Development Institute, 2012.

[38] Tun W, Okal J, Schenk K, Esantsi S, Mutale F, Kyeremaa RK, et al. Limited accessibility to HIV services for persons with disabilities living with HIV in Ghana, Uganda and Zambia. J Int AIDS Soc 2016;19(5 Suppl 4).

[39] Ingstad B, Whyte SR. Disability and culture: Berkeley, CA: University California Press, 1995.

[40] Hoogeveen JG. Measuring welfare for small but vulnerable groups: Poverty and disability in Uganda. J Afr Econ 2005;14(4):603-31.

[41] Foley D, Chowdhury J. Poverty, social exclusion and the politics of disability: Care as a social good and the expenditure of social capital in Chuadanga, Bangladesh. Soc Policy Adm 2007;41(4):372-85.

In: Disability: International Aspects
Editors: Ariel Tenenbaum et al.
ISBN: 978-1-53617-886-9

Chapter 5

FISCAL VALUE OF DISABILITY-ADJUSTED-LIFE-YEARS LOST IN THE ECONOMIC AND MONETARY COMMUNITY OF CENTRAL AFRICA (CEMAC)

Joses M Kirigia*, PhD, MA, BEd,
Rose NDK Muthuri, MA, BA
and Newton G Muthuri, BBA
African Sustainable Development Research Consortium (ASDRC), Nairobi, Kenya

ABSTRACT

The Economic and Monetary Community of Central Africa (CEMAC) consists of Cameroon, Central African Republic, Chad, Republic of Congo, Equatorial Guinea and Gabon. In 2015, CEMAC lost a total of 38,356,492 disability-adjusted-life-years (DALY). This study estimated

* Corresponding Author: Joses Muthuri Kirigia, PhD, Associate Professor of Health Economics, African Sustainable Development Research Consortium (ASDRC), POBox 6994 00100 GPO, Nairobi, Kenya. E-mail: kirigiajoses@gmail.com.

the fiscal value of DALYs lost in the CEMAC in 2015 without and with the UN Sustainable Development Goal 3. The fiscal value of DALYs lost from each cause (disease) in each CEMAC member state was estimated by multiplying DALYs lost by GDP per person net of health expenditures. The 38,356,492 DALYs lost in CEMAC in 2015 had a fiscal value of Int$140,106,558,107. Approximately 61.3% of CEMAC's total fiscal value of DALYs lost was caused by communicable, maternal, perinatal and nutritional conditions; 28.4% by non-communicable diseases; and 10.3% by injuries. Cameroon sustained 36.6% of the total fiscal value of DALYs, Central African Republic 2.0%, Chad 24.4%, Republic of Congo 10.5%, Equatorial Guinea 15.5%, and Gabon 11.0%. The CEMAC sub-region could save about 31.8% of the total fiscal value of DALYs lost if SDG 3 targets 3.1, 3.2, 3.3, 3.4 and 3.6 are fully achieved. Thus, CEMAC member states should make sufficient investment into national systems that tackle determinants of health to ensure universal coverage of pertinent services, and ultimately, attain SDG3 on ensuring healthy lives and promotion of well-being for all people at all ages. These kinds of studies should be complemented with economic evaluations of alternative preventive, curative and rehabilitative interventions into diseases to guide priority setting, health policy development and decision-making in CEMAC.

ABBREVIATIONS

AIDS	Acquired Immune Deficiency Syndrome
AMU	Arab Maghreb Union
AU	African Union
CBA	Cost Benefit Analysis
CEMAC	Economic and Monetary Community of Central Africa
CFVD	Country's Fiscal Value of DALYs
CHE	Current Health Expenditure
COI	Cost-of-Illness
CMPN	Communicable, maternal, perinatal and nutritional conditions
CV	Contingent Valuation Approach
DALY	Disability-Adjusted-Life-Year
$DALY_{0\text{-}4}$	Discounted total DALYs lost to the jth disease among people aged 0–4 years

$DALY_{5-14}$	Discounted total DALYs lost to the jth disease among people aged 5–14 years
$DALY_{15-29}$	Discounted total DALYs lost to the jth disease among people aged 15–29 years
$DALY_{30-49}$	Discounted total DALYs lost to the jth disease among people aged 30–49 years
$DALY_{50-59}$	Discounted total DALYs lost to the jth disease among people aged 50–59 years
$DALY_{60-69}$	Discounted total DALYs lost to the jth disease among people aged 60–69 years
$DALY_{70+}$	Discounted total DALYs lost to the jth disease among people aged 70 years and above
EAC	East African Community
FVD	Fiscal Value of DALY
FVD_{0-4}	Fiscal value of DALYs lost among people aged 0-4 years
FVD_{5-14}	Fiscal value of DALYs lost among people aged 5-14 years
FVD_{15-29}	Fiscal value of DALYs lost among people aged 15-29 years
FVD_{30-49}	Fiscal value of DALYs lost among people aged 30-49 years
FVD_{50-59}	Fiscal value of DALYs lost among people aged 50-59 years
FVD_{60-69}	Fiscal value of DALYs lost among people aged 60-69 years
$FVD_{=>70}$	Fiscal value of DALYs lost among people aged 70 years and above
GDP	Gross Domestic Product
$GDPPC_{Int\$}$	GDP per capita in Purchasing Power Parity
HCA	Human Capital Approach
HIV	Human Immunodeficiency Virus
INJ:	Injury
Int$	International Dollar or Purchasing Power Parity (PPP)
MNCH	Maternal new born and child health
NCD	Non-Communicable Disease

$NHGDPPC_{Int\$}$	Per capita non-health GDP in PPP
NTD	Neglected Tropical Disease
OECD	Organisation for Economic Co-operation and Development
SDG	Sustainable Development Goal
UHC	Universal Health Coverage
UN	United Nations Organization
UNGA	United Nations General Assembly
US$	United States of America Dollar
TB	Tuberculosis
TFVD	Total Fiscal Value of Total DALYs
WHO	World Health Organization
WTA	Willing to Accept
WTP	Willingness to Pay

INTRODUCTION

The Economic and Monetary Community of Central Africa (CEMAC) consists of Cameroon, Central African Republic, Chad, Republic of Congo, Equatorial Guinea and Gabon (1). CEMAC has a total population of 49.7 million people. Its total gross domestic product was Int$ 235.74 billion in 2018; and per capita GDP of Int$ 4,748 (STD= 12,437) (2).

In 2015, CEMAC lost a total of 38,356,492 disability-adjusted-life-years (DALY) [3]. Approximately, 24.6 million (64%) DALY were lost from communicable, maternal, perinatal and nutritional conditions; 9.8 million (26%) were from non-communicable diseases; and 3.9 million (10%) were from injuries. The heavy disease burden is attributed to sub-optimally performing national health systems (4-6), other systems that meet other basic needs (e.g., education, food, shelter, water, sanitation, security) (7) and national research for health systems (8).

The weakness of national health systems is clearly manifested in the sub-optimal universal health coverage (UHC) service index of 44% in Cameroon, 33% in Central African Republic, 29% in Chad, 38% in

Republic of Congo, 45% in Equatorial Guinea and 52% in Gabon (9). The index includes reproductive, maternal, new-born and child health, infectious diseases, non-communicable diseases and service capacity and access. Thus, Cameroon, Central African Republic, Chad, Congo, Equatorial Guinea and Gabon health services coverage fall short of the optimal performance by 56%, 67%, 71%, 62%, 55%, and 48% percentage points respectively. As shown in table 1, the CEMAC member states health service coverage gap is attributed to low densities of health workers, health infrastructure and technologies compared to global averages (9, 10).

Table 1. Health systems indicators for Economic and Monetary Community of Central Africa (CEMAC) Member States

Health System Indicators	**Cameroon**	**Central African Republic**	**Chad**	**Republic of Congo**	**Equatorial Guinea**	**Gabon**	**Global average**
Physicians per 10000 population*	0.8	0.5	-	1	-	-	13.9
Nursing and midwifery personnel per 10000 population*	4.4	2.6	-	8.2	-	-	28.6
Dentistry personnel per 10000 population*-0	<0.05	<0.05	-	-	-	-	2.8
-Pharmaceutical personnel per 10000 population*	<0.05	<0.05	-	0.2	-	-	4.5
Psychiatrists per 10000 population*		<0.05	-	<0.05	-	-	0.2
Hospitals per 100000 population*	0.8	0.5	0.7	-	-	3.5	-
Psychiatric beds per 100 000 population*	-	0.7	-	0.9	-	-	22.9
Computed tomography units per million population*	0.6	0.0	0.1	-	-	3.6	-
Radiotherapy units per million population*	0.1	0.0	-	-	-	0.6	1.8
Mammography Units per million population*	17.4	4.7	4.7	-	-	74.1	-
Current Health Expenditure (CHE) per Capita in US$ (2015)**	64	17	36	59	280	198	822

Source: *WHO (10), **WHO (9).

The low health systems inputs densities emanate from the fact that current health expenditures per capita for CEMAC member states of between US$ 17 and US$280 (9) are lower than the US$74 to US$984 per person recommended for attainment of United Nations (UN) Sustainable Development Goal 3 (SDG3) (11). Economic valuations of health losses have been calculated and fruitfully used in Arab Maghreb Union (12), Asian (13), East African Community (14), European (15), North American (16, 17), and South American countries (18) to advocate for increased investments into health development.

To date, no study has estimated the financial value of DALYs lost from a wide range of diseases and conditions in the CEMAC sub-region. Thus, aim of this study is to contribute to bridging that knowledge gap. The specific objectives were: (a) to estimate the financial value of DALYs lost in the CEMAC in 2015 without SDGs; (b) to estimate the reductions in financial value of DALY losses assuming some of SDG 3 targets are attained by 2030; and (c) to review briefly the recent health SDG-related resolutions adopted by the United Nations General Assembly (UNGA), which if fully implemented could fast-track achievement of SDG 3 targets in CEMAC sub-region.

LITERATURE REVIEW

In the extant literature, two main approaches have been used in the fiscal valuation of health outcomes (e.g., health-related quality of life, health-adjusted-life-expectancy, quality-adjusted-life-year, disability-adjusted-life-yea, life expectancy, statistical life), i.e., the willingness-to-pay (WTP) approach and the human capital approach (HCA).

Willingness-to-Pay Approach

The French engineer cum economist pioneered monetary measurement of utility from public projects, e.g., roads. According to Dupuit "…the measure of the utility of an object [is] the maximum sacrifice which each consumer would be willing to make in order to acquire the object" (19). Schelling (20) helped clarify that the relevant valuation concept was people's willingness to trade off money for small risks. Thus, in the context of the current study, if the WTP approach were to be used, the value of a DALY lost can be measured either as the maximum amount of money a CEMAC citizen would be willing to pay (WTP) in order to avert the risk of losing a statistical DALY or the minimum amount of money a CEMAC citizen would be willing to accept (WTA) for incurring the risk of losing a DALY (21). Studies have found that WTA values are far much higher than WTP values (22); which has been attributed to endowment effects and loss aversion (23). The WTP values are usually elicited using contingent valuation approach, where people are asked directly in a survey how much money they would be willing to sacrifice for a clearly defined health outcome, health service, health intervention or health system input. According to Russel, Fox-Rushby and Arhin (24), a WTP survey questionnaire should have four components: (a) past health care practices, expenditure and attitudes; (b) creation of a plausible hypothetical market; (c). questions which elicit the respondents' willingness and ability to pay for health service on offer; and (d) questions about the respondents' or household's characteristics.

In a survey for eliciting WTP values for averting DALY loss, not all four components would be applicable for a number of reasons. First, it's unlikely that respondents will have had past experience of trading off money for risk aversion of DALY loss. Second, since DALY is a non-traded commodity, construction of a plausible hypothetical market, might be problematic because it would be challenging (a) for respondents, majority of whom are illiterate or semi-literate in CEMAC context, to understand what a DALY means; (b) to develop convincing organizational set-up within which DALYs will be traded; (c) to develop realistic method of payment; (d) to explain effectiveness of health intervention that would save the said DALY, given the uncertainty in medicine; and (e) an individual's WTP for safety improvement will presumably reflect his aversion to the adverse consequences of death or injury (25-27).

The WTP (or contingent valuation) has been applied to value statistical lives in Sweden (28) and USA (27); road safety improvement to reduce risk of non-fatal physical injuries in France (29); WTP for a reduction in road-mortality risk in Sweden (30); WTP for risk reduction of traffic accidents and time saved in Europe (31); WTP for risk reduction of traffic accidents and time saved in North Cyprus (32); monetary valuations for programme benefits for use in cost-benefit analysis (CBA) (33); monetary valuation of cardiovascular disease in Canada (34); and contingent valuation (CV) of WTP for mortality risk reduction in Ontario (35).

In Africa the contingent valuation survey approach has been used to elicit WTP for health insurance in the informal sector of Sierra Leone (36); community-based health insurance in Burkina Faso (37), Cameroon (38), Ethiopia (39), Ghana (40) and Nigeria (41, 42). The contingent valuation approach has also been used to elicit WTP for National Health Insurance Fund in Nigeria (43, 44); national health insurance in South Sudan (45); healthcare in public health facilities in Uganda (46); improved malaria treatment programme in Zambia (47); artemisinin-based combination therapy in rural Tanzania (48); praziquantel treatment in a hyperendemic community of Ogun State, Nigeria (49); and condoms in Kenya, Nigeria, South Africa, Zambia, and Zimbabwe (50). In addition, Ternent et al. (51) elicited WTP for maternal health outcomes in Burkina Faso; and Kirigia et al. (52) elicited WTP for schistosomiasis-related health outcomes.

A few of the advantages of WTP approach are that it values the relevant concept of reduction in the probability of statistical death and/or morbidity (20); explicitly incorporates people's current preferences (53); consistency with the Potential Pareto Improvement Criterion, which requires beneficiaries of a health policy change (or project) could hypothetically compensate the losers from the change and still be better off (54, 55); its rooted in economic welfare theory of utility maximization and consumer sovereignty (56); externalities or spillover effects (positive or negative) can be captured (57); it can be used to value changes in both life expectancy and health-related quality of life; and politically appealing because individual citizen preferences counts (58).

Some of the disadvantages of WTP approach include: individuals WTP values depend on wealth/income (i.e., ability to pay) (56), and their use in valuation of health outcome would give disproportionate weight to preferences to relatively affluent segment of the population; WTP hypothetical trade-offs are not validated (56); and respondents may not reveal their true preferences due to either strategic response or social desirability effects (59); WTP has been found not to increase with the quantity of the consumed good, implying lack of or inadequate scope effect (60, 61). Smith and Sachs (62) throw the following caution:

> "CV does not seem to be capitalising on the major advantages it holds as a technique over other outcome methodologies. Overall, it is unclear why and how a decision maker could use existing CV studies in resource allocation decision-making. This failure to capitalise on the potential advantages of CV by researchers could suggest that training in the technique is inadequate, the technique is fundamentally flawed, the costs of doing CV appropriately are astronomical, or simply that there are inadequate guidelines available to guide researchers" (62).

Human Capital Approach

The Organisation for Economic Co-operation and Development (OECD) (63) defined human capital as "The [health], knowledge, skills, competencies and attitudes embodied in individuals that facilitate the creation of personal, social and economic wellbeing" (p. 18). Lundvall and Johnson (64) delineates four categories of knowledge: (a) know-what referring to possession of facts; (b) know-why denotes scientific knowledge of principles and laws of motion in nature, human mind and society; (c) know-who (when and where) refers to specific and selective social relations, e.g., knowledge of markets, target populations for public health intervention, professional networks, learning communities, communities of practice, and professional associations; (d) know-how referring to skills, i.e., technical ability or expertise of performing specific activities or tasks well, e.g., diagnosis of infections, treatments. We concur with the authors that innovation of health system, health care delivery models, health interventions, health products, norms and standards entails judicious combination of these four categories of knowledge by an entrepreneur. According to OECD (63) human capital is developed during the entire person's life-course in the context of conception, birth and growing up within community, family and household settings; formal education and training; work place training (research and development, seminars, workshops, conferences, webinars); and informal learning on-the-job.

Premature death, from whatever cause, means a permanent loss of health stock, knowledge, skills, and competencies hitherto embodied in the disease (or injury) victim. Non-fatal morbidity from disease and injuries causes temporary erosion of stock of human capital, and hence, capability of performing societal functions or roles. Arguably, a disability-adjusted-life-year (DALY) is a non-monetary proxy measure of attrition in human capital, i.e., the time lived with a disability and the time lost due to premature mortality (65).

Weisbrod (66) attempted to develop a framework for estimating the value of the stock of human capital. He viewed the value of a person in terms of his/her worth as a productive asset in society. The author explains that valuation of a person can potentially be done in two ways. One, if definition of society includes the person being valued, a measure of value as gross productivity, without deducting his consumption would be relevant. In this case, according to Weisbrod (66), the gross present value of a man (the present value of expected future earnings) at a given age would be obtained by multiplying value of output during each year of age, the probabilities of surviving to each age, and the discount factor. Two, if definition of society does not include the person being valued, there would be need to deduct his consumption from gross productivity to obtain net productivity. Weisbrod (66) used computed present values of gross future earnings of United States males by age in 1950 by multiplying each age group's mean money earnings per year by percent employed, probability of surviving through a year, and discount factor. He obtained net future earnings through multiplication of each age group's mean money earnings per year by percent of persons employed minus value of consumption; and then multiplying the answer by probability of surviving through a year, and discount factor.

The HCA methods developed by Weisbrod (66) have been applied globally to value productivity losses attributed to non-fatal disability and premature mortality from various causes. Some examples of HCA applications in the United States include Robinson and Hammitt (67) review of studies that valued reductions in fatal illness risks in the United States that yielded estimates varying from $4.2 million to $13.7 million (with a mid-point of $9.0 million) per statistical life in 2013 dollars.

Hurd et al. (68) estimated the total annual societal cost of dementia in USA at between US$159 billion (from cost of forgone wages approach) and $215 billion (from replacement cost approach) in 2010. Out of the latter, US$124 billion was attributed to productivity losses related to premature mortality and US$77 billion were direct medical costs. They found the total annual societal cost per case to be between US$41,000 to US$56,000.

DeVol and Bedroussian (69) analysed the economic cost of seven of the most common chronic Diseases (cancer, diabetes, hypertension, stroke, heart disease, pulmonary conditions, and mental disorders) in the United States. Their analysis revealed United States incurred a total economic loss of US$1.3 trillion annually; which was made up of $1.1 trillion (79.9%) per year from lost productivity and $277 billion (20.1%) spent on health system-related treatment costs. The authors estimated that improvements in chronic diseases prevention and treatment may avert 40 million cases leading an increase in GDP of $905 billion from productivity gains and a decrease in treatment costs of $218 billion per year.

Rice, Hodgson and Kopstein (17) estimated the economic burden of illness, disability and premature death from all causes in the United States in 1980 to be US$ 415.92 billion. This was made up of US$211,143 million (51%) of direct cost; US$67,827 million (16%) of productivity losses from morbidity; and US$136,948 million (33%) from premature mortality.

The Public Health Agency of Canada (16), using a prevalence-based cost-of-illness (COI) study, found the total cost of disease and injury in Canada to be $18.7 billion in 2010. That cost was made up of total value of production lost due to morbidity of $18.2 billion (97.5%); and $ 463.5 million (2.5%) from premature mortality.

We also refer to a few examples of HCA applications in South America. Castaneda-Orjuela et al. (70) using a dynamic transmission model predicted there were 35,739 cases of dengue in 2011; 988 (2.8%) of them had severe dengue; and 102 died of dengue in Colombia. The authors estimated total nationwide cost of dengue prevention and control was between US$54 million and US$56 million nationwide. Out of which, US$16.9 million (CI 95% 15.2–18.5 million) consisted of health care cost of managing dengue and between US$37 and US$42 million annual cost of vector control.

Laserna, Barahona-Correa, Baquero, Castañeda-Cardona and Rosselli (18) conducted a systematic review of the economic impact studies of dengue fever conducted in Latin America and the Caribbean. The authors found the average annual cost was more than US$ 3 billion; with about 80% consisting of productivity losses.

Bloom, Chen and McGovern (71) analyses the macroeconomic impact of noncommunicable diseases (NCDs) and mental health conditions in Costa Rica, Jamaica, and Peru. The authors found cost of all NCDs and mental health conditions to be US$ 81.96 billion (US$ 16 143 per capita) for cost Costa Rica, US$ 18.45 billion (US$ 6 306 per capita) for Jamaica and US$ 477.33 billion (US$ 15 010 per capita) for Peru in 2015.

We also review a few examples of HCA applications in Europe. Olesen, Gustavsson, Svensson, Wittchen and Jonsson (72) estimated annual costs for 19 mental and neurologic disorders in 30 European countries in 2010. They found the total cost of brain disorders to be €798 billion. The average cost per person with a brain disorder varied between €285 for headache and €30 000 for neuromuscular disorders.

Luengo-Fernandez, Leal, Gray and Sullivan (15) estimated that cancer costed 27 countries of the European Union €126 billion, which was made up of €51.0 billion (40.4%) of health care costs, €42.6 billion (33.8%) of productivity losses from mortality, €9.43 billion (7.4%) from morbidity, and €23.2 billion (18.4%) of informal care cost in 2009.

Luengo-Fernandez, Leal, Gray, Petersen and Rayner (73) estimated the cost of cardiovascular diseases in the United Kingdom to be £29.11 billion in 2004. The total cost consisted of health care cost of £17,386.19 (59.7%); informal care by economically active and non-active carers cost of £5,065.78 (13.6%); productivity losses associated premature mortality costed £3,945.25 (13.6%); and productivity losses associated with morbidity costed £2,716.53 (9.3%).

Liu, Maniadakis, Gray and Rayner (74) using human capital approach estimated the total cost of coronary heart disease in the UK in 1999 to be £7.06 billion; which consists of £1,730.07 million (25%) of direct health care cost; £2,908.71 million (41%) of productivity loss from premature mortality and morbidity; and 2,416.51 million (34%) of informal care (time of economically active and inactive caregivers).

We also give a few examples of HCA application in South-East Asia. Acharya, Rau, Udupa, Rajan and Vijayanarayana (13) evaluated the COI (cost of treatment, investigation, consultation fee, intervention cost, transportation, days lost due to work, and hospitalization) for diabetic inpatients in medical wards of Kasturba tertiary care hospital with or without complications. The authors found annual total COI of diabetes care per patient without complication was 22,456.97 Rupees; 30,634.45 Rupees per diabetes patient with complications; 164,211.40 Rupees per diabetes patient with complications and on dialysis; and 166,785.85 Rupees per diabetes patient with complications and on cardiac intervention.

According to Collins, Hafidz and Mustikawati (75) estimated the total economic cost treating TB cases in Indonesia to be US$ 6,955,177,790 in 2015. This consists of provider medical costs of $156,233,136 (2.2%); patient out-of-pocket costs of $74,967,714 (1.1%); productivity losses due to illness of $700,847,370 (10.1%); and productivity losses due to premature death of $6,023,129,571 (86.6%).

Pitayatienanan et al. (76) estimated total cost of obesity in Thailand at 12,142 million baht (725.3 million Int$, 16.74 baht =1 Int$). It consisted of 5,584 million baht (46.0%) of health care cost; 5,864 million baht (48.3%)

of productivity losses associated with premature mortality; and 694 million baht (5.7%) of productivity losses from morbidity.

Ranaweera et al. (77), using the WHO gross costing approach, estimated the present value of economic cost of selected alcohol related disease conditions in Sri Lanka in 2015 at US$ 885.86 million. It composed of direct cost of US$ 388.35 million (43.8%) and indirect cost of US$ 497.50 million (56.2%). The road traffic injuries resulted in economic losses of US$ 251.28 million (28.4%), which were made up of direct health care cost of US$116.31 million (46.3%), morbidity-related absenteeism productivity losses of US$56.66 million (22.5%), and premature mortality-related indirect cost of US$ 78.30 million (31.2%).

Amarasinghe et al. (78) estimated tobacco-related cancers cost of illness in Sri Lanka in 2015 to be to be US$121.2 million; which composed of direct cost of US$42.1 million (34.7%) and indirect cost of US$79.1 million (65.3%). Cancer of the lip, oral cavity and pharynx accounted for 34% of the direct cost; and cancer of the trachea, lung and bronchus was responsible for 41% of the indirect cost.

The HCA has also been applied in Western Pacific. Xu, Wang, Wimo, Fratiglioni and Qiu (79) estimated and projected the costs of dementia in China for the periods 1990–2010 and 2020–2030. According to the authors total cost of dementia increased from US$ 0.9 billion in 1990 to US$ 47.2 billion in 2010; and projected it to reach US$ 69.0 billion by 2020 and US$ 114.2 billion by 2030.

Hayata et al. (80) used the COI method to estimate the direct and indirect costs associated with cervical cancer in Japan in 1996 to 2011 to make predictions for 2014 to 2020. The study found that COI increased from 96.1 billion yen in 1996 to 159.9 billion yen in 2011, i.e., a 66.4% increase. The 1996 total COI was made up of direct health system cost of 15.8 billion Yen (16%), morbidity-related productivity losses of 10.4 billion Yen (11%), and premature mortality productivity losses of 69.9 billion Yen (73%). The projected total COI was 159.5 billion yen in 2014 and 156.8 billion yen in 2020, i.e., a 1.7% decrease.

Peabody, Shimkhada, Tan and Luck (81) estimated that nationally tuberculosis costed the Philippines a total of between US$153 million to

US$174 million in 1997. About 19.8% of latter is made up of annual loss due to mortality; 63.6% due to morbidity; and 16.7% due to treatment of all TB cases.

Finally, we refer to a few examples of HCA applications in the African Region. Kirigia and Mwabu (14) employing HCA appraised monetary value of 82,017,651 DALYs lost in 2015 in the East African Community (EAC) in 2015 to be Int$203,843,476,166. They assessed the average monetary value per DALY lost at Int$ 2,485; ranging between a minimum of Int$764 in Burundi and a maximum of Int$ 3,167 in Kenya.

Muthuri, Muthuri and Kirigia (12) evaluated the total pecuniary value of DALYs lost in the Arab Maghreb Union (AMU) in 2016 at Int$ 289,033,271,814. They found average pecuniary value per DALY lost was Int$ 10,636, and varied from a minimum of Int$ 4226 in Mauritania to a maximum of Int$ 13,852 in Algeria.

Kirigia et al. (82) used HCA to estimate the non-health GDP losses associated with NCD deaths in the WHO African Region. The authors estimated that the 2,788,381 NCD deaths that occurred in the African Region in 2012 resulted in a total discounted non-health GDP loss of Int$ 61,302,450,005. The regional average non-health GDP loss was Int$ 21,985 per NCD death. The average non-health GDP loss of Int$ 54,534 per NCD death in high and upper middle income group was 2.5-fold that of lower middle-income group and 6.0-fold that of low income group of the African Region countries.

Kirigia and Mburugu (83) estimated value of 67,860 human lives lost in 2015 due to NTDs at Int$ 5,112,472,607; of which 14.6% was incurred by high and upper middle income countries, 57.7% by lower middle income countries, and 27.7% by lower income continental Africa countries. The continental mean value of human life lost was Int$ 75,339 per NTD death. The average value of human life lost among high-income and upper middle-income countries of Int$ 231,278 was 2-fold and 6-fold that of lower middle-income countries and low-income countries respectively.

The HCA has been widely used due to its simplicity and also because the necessary data on mortality and earnings are readily available (84, 85).

Various authors have pointed out a number of drawbacks of the HCA: inconsistence with economics potential Pareto improvement criterion (86); singular focus on the dead and the sick vis-à-vis the living members of society (87, 88); it ignores the existence of caring externality (89), participation utility (90), altruism (91), and religious externality (21); it measures livelihood rather than health per se (92); it completely ignores potential beneficiaries preferences (93, 94); and if applied in CEMAC without adjustment it would discriminate against housewives (whose output is not captured in GDP calculations), the retired, the children, the handicapped, and the unemployed (95). We concur with critiques that HCA estimates should never be used to set health priorities, since they do not reflect cost and benefits of alternative interventions (96) into diseases. The estimates from HCA should be used purely for public health advocacy, i.e., to raise awareness of potential impact of disease on present value of future economic output.

The study reported in this article applied HCA because necessary data on per capita health expenditure, per capita GDP, and DALYs for a wide array of diseases were available for all CEMAC member states.

OUR STUDY

This study used the conceptual framework developed and applied in estimating the money value of DALYs lost in the EAC (14), the AMU (12) and Kenya (97). The EAC, AMU and Kenya studies applied HCA to convert DALY lost into their money equivalents. As recommended first by Weisbrod (66), and subsequently, by WHO (98) we deducted consumption from gross productivity to obtain net productivity.

The CEMAC total fiscal value of total DALYs (TFVD) lost from all causes is the sum of each of the six country's fiscal value of DALYs (CFVD) lost from all causes (12, 14):

$$TFVD = \sum_{country=1}^{country=6} \{CFVD_i\}. \tag{1}$$

Where i= Cameroon, Central African Republic, Chad, Republic of Congo, Equatorial Guinea and Gabon.

Following Kirigia, Mburugu and Huka (97), Kirigia and Mwabu (14) and Muthuri, Muthuri and Kirigia (12), we estimated each country's CFVD lost due to the jth disease as the sum of fiscal value of DALYs lost among people aged 0-4 years (FVD_{0-4}), 5-14 years (FVD_{5-14}), 15-29 years 15-29 years (FVD_{15-29}), 30-49 years (FVD_{30-49}), 50-59 years (FVD_{50-59}), 60-69 years (FVD_{60-69}), and 70 years and above ($FVD_{=>70}$). The FVD associated with the jth disease DALYs lost among people of a specific age group are the product of the per capita non-health GDP in purchasing power parity (PPP) and the total jth disease DALYs lost within a specific age group (12, 14, 97).

Each ith country's discounted total FVD attributable to the jth disease DALYs were estimated using equations 2 through 9 below (12, 14, 97).

$$\sum_{0-4}^{\geq 70}(CFVD_{0-4} + CFVD_{5-14} + CFVD_{15-29} + .. + CFVD_{=>70}). \tag{2}$$

$$CFVD_{0-4} = [NHGDPPC_{Int\$}] \times [DALY_{0-4}]\} \tag{3}$$

$$CFVD_{5-14} = [NHGDPPC_{Int\$}] \times [DALY_{5-14}]\} \tag{4}$$

$$CFVD_{15-29} = [NHGDPPC_{Int\$}] \times [DALY_{15-29}]\} \tag{5}$$

$$CFVD_{30-49} = [NHGDPPC_{Int\$}] \times [DALY_{30-49}]\}. \tag{6}$$

$$CFVD_{50-59} = [NHGDPPC_{Int\$}] \times [DALY_{50-59}]\}. \tag{7}$$

$$CFVD_{60-69} = [NHGDPPC_{Int\$}] \times [DALY_{60-69}]\} \tag{8}$$

$$CFVD_{\geq 70} = [NHGDPPC_{Int\$}] \times [DALY_{\geq 70}]\} \quad (9)$$

Where: $NHGDPPC_{Int\$}$ is the per capita non-health GDP in purchasing power parity (PPP), which was obtained by subtracting the per capita total health expenditure from the per capita GDP ($GDPPC_{Int\$}$); $DALY_{0-4}$, $DALY_{5-14}$, $DALY_{15-29}$, $DALY_{30-49}$, $DALY_{50-59}$, $DALY_{60-69}$ and $DALY_{70+}$ are the discounted total DALYs lost to the jth disease among people aged 0–4 years, 5–14 years, 15–29 years, 30–49 years, 50–59 years, 60–69 years, and 70 years and above in country $_i$ in 2015 (12, 14, 97).

Estimation of the Reductions in Fiscal Value of DALY Losses in CEMAC Assuming SDG 3 Related Targets Are Achieved

Table 2 reproduces the United Nations Sustainable Development Goal 3 targets.

The reductions in CEMAC fiscal values of DALYs lost assuming the SDG3 targets for maternal mortality ratio (Target 3.1), neonatal mortality (Target 3.2), children under 5 years of age mortality (Target 3.2), and HIV/AIDS deaths (Target 3.3) are achieved were estimated using the following equation (12, 14):

$$FVD_{HCj2030} = \sum_{Country=1}^{Country=5} \left\{ FVD_{HCj2015} - \left[FVD_{HCj2015} \times \frac{HCj2015 - SDG_{jHCT}}{HCj2015} \right] \right\}$$

Where: $FVD_{HCj2030}$ is the total fiscal value of DALYs expected to be lost in CEMAC from jth health condition in 2030 assuming related target is fully achieved; $FVD_{HCj2015}$ is the total pecuniary value of DALYs actually lost in CEMAC from jth health condition in baseline year 2015; HC_{j2015} is the jth health condition target mortality rate in 2015; HC_{j2030} is the jth health condition target mortality rate in 2030; and SDG_{jHCT} is the SDG jth health condition target mortality rate (12).

Table 2. Targets envisaged in UN SDG 3

Target	Description	Percentage reduction envisaged in SDG targets
SDG 3.1	By 2030, reduce the global maternal mortality ratio to less than 70 per 100,000 live births (9, 99).	88%
SDG 3.2	By 2030, end preventable deaths of newborns, with all countries aiming to reduce neonatal mortality to at least as low as 12 per 1,000 live births (99).	59%
SDG 3.3	By 2030, end the epidemics of AIDS, tuberculosis, malaria and neglected tropical diseases and reduce hepatitis, water-borne diseases and other communicable diseases (99).	
	(a). Reduce global HIV-related deaths from 1,062,352 in 2015 to below 500,000 by 2020 (100).	53%
	(b). Malaria mortality rates will be reduced globally by at least 90% from 2015 to 2030 (101).	90%
	The number of tuberculosis (TB) deaths will be reduced by 90% from 2015 to 2030 (102).	90%
	Mortality due to vector-borne diseases will be reduced globally by at least 75% from 2016 to 2030 (103).	75%
SDG 3.4	By 2030, reduce premature mortality due to NCDs by one third through prevention and treatment and promote mental health and well-being (99).	33.3%
SDG 3.6	By 2020, halve the number of global deaths and injuries from road traffic accidents (99).	50%

Sources: Targets in Table 2 were obtained from UN (99), WHO (9), WHO (100), WHO (101), WHO (102), WHO and (103).

The reductions in CEMAC fiscal values of DALYs lost assuming the SDG3 targets for death associated with tuberculosis (Target 3.3), malaria (Target 3.3), neglected tropical diseases (NTD) (Target 3.3), NCD (Target 3.4), and injuries (Target 3.6) are attained were estimated using the following equation (12):

$$FVD_{HCj2030} = \sum_{Country=1}^{Country=5} \{FVD_{HCj2015} - [FVD_{HCj2015} \times SDG_{jHCT}]\}$$

Data source and software

The nine equations in preceding subsection were estimated using Excel Software developed by Microsoft (New York). The per capita total health expenditure data were from the WHO Global Health Expenditure Database (104), per capita GDP data from the International Monetary Fund World Economic Outlook database (2), and DALYs data from the WHO Global Health Observatory (3).

Ethics Approval

Ethical approval and consent to participate was not applicable for the study reported in this manuscript. This is because it did not involve the use of any animal or human data or products. It was based sorely on secondary statistical data published in the International Monetary Fund and World Health Organization websites.

FINDINGS

In 2015, CEMAC lost a total of 38,356,492 DALYs from all causes with a fiscal value of Int$ 140,106,558,107 (see Table 3). About 36.6% of the total fiscal value of DALYs lost was borne by Cameroon, 2.0% by Central African Republic, 24.4% by Chad, 10.5% by the Republic of Congo, 15.6% by Equatorial Guinea, and 11.0% by Gabon. Thus, Cameroon and Chad alone accounted for 61% of the total fiscal value of DALYs lost in CEMAC.

Approximately Int$ 85,877,934,976 (61.3%) of CEMAC's total fiscal value of DALYs lost was caused by communicable, maternal, perinatal and nutritional conditions (CMPN); Int$ 39,819,229,718 (28.4%) by non-communicable diseases (NCD); and Int$ 14,409,393,413 (10.3%) by injuries (INJ).

Almost 52.6% of the fiscal value of CMPN DALY loss was from infectious and parasitic diseases; 17.7% from respiratory infectious; 2.8% from maternal conditions; 20.3% from neonatal conditions; and 6.6% from nutritional deficiencies. Figure 1 shows fiscal value of DALYs lost from infectious and parasitic diseases in CEMAC. HIV/AIDS, diarrhoeal diseases, malaria and meningitis accounted for 73% of the fiscal value of DALYs lost from infectious and parasitic diseases.

Table 3. Financial value of DALYs lost from all causes in CEMAC member states (Int$ or PPP, in 2015)

Country	(A). DALYS in 2015*	(B). Total Financial Value of DALY (Int$)**	(C). Population*	(D=B/C). Financial Value per person in population (Int$)**	(E=B/A). Financial Value per DALY (Int$)**
Cameroon	16,351,407	51,321,465,764	23,345,000	2,198	3,139
Central African Republic	4,537,291	2,838,481,756	4,831,000	588	626
Chad	13,791,728	34,225,426,775	14,055,000	2,435	2,482
Congo	2,282,734	14,655,518,776	4,622,000	3,171	6,420
Equatorial Guinea	579,409	21,784,894,414	866,000	25,156	37,598
Gabon	813,923	15,280,770,622	1,745,000	8,757	18,774
TOTAL	38,356,492	140,106,558,107	49,464,000	2,832	3,653

Source: *Statistics from WHO (3). **Results from authors calculations.

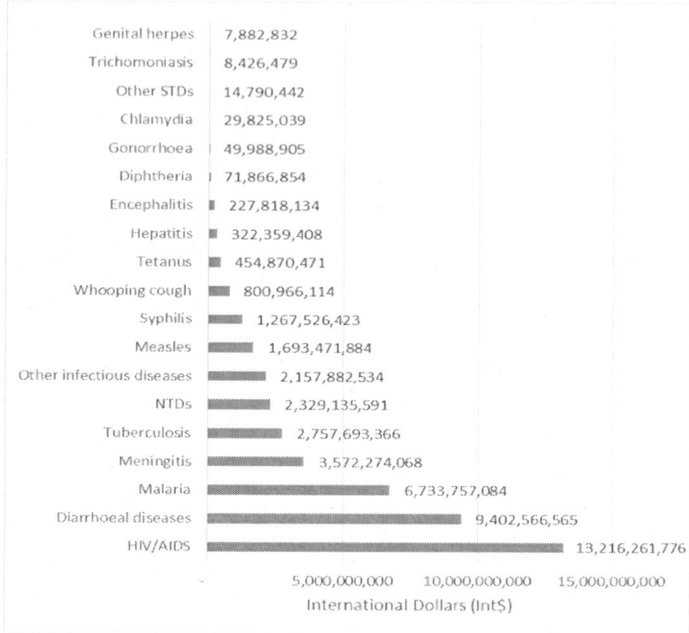

Source: Authors estimates.

Figure 1. Fiscal value of DALY losses from infectious and parasitic diseases in CEMAC (2015 Int$ or PPP).

Figure 2 portrays fiscal value of DALYs lost from respiratory infections, maternal conditions, neonatal conditions and nutritional deficiencies in CEMAC. About 98% of the Int$ 15.2 billion fiscal value of DALY loss from respiratory infections was caused by lower respiratory infections. Out of the Int$17.4 billion of neonatal conditions related DALYs lost resulted from preterm birth complications (39.2%), birth asphyxia and birth trauma (37.6%), neonatal sepsis and infections (17.1%), and other neonatal conditions (6.0%).

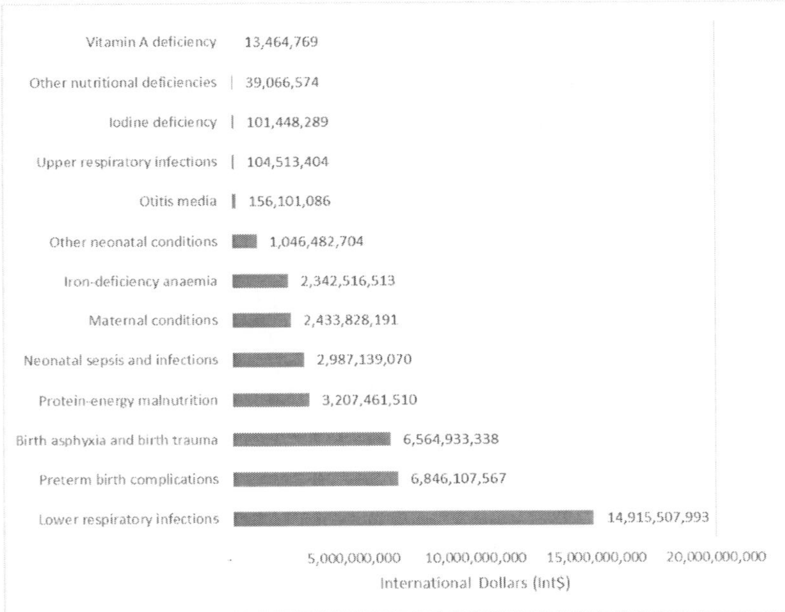

Source: Authors estimates.

Figure 2. Fiscal value of DALYs lost from respiratory infections, maternal conditions, neonatal conditions and nutritional deficiencies in CEMAC (2015 Int$ or PPP).

Approximately 56.2% of the Int$ 5.7 billion fiscal value of DALYs lost from nutritional deficiencies was caused by protein-energy malnutrition; 41.1% by iron-deficiency anaemia; 1.8% by iodine deficiency; 0.2% by vitamin A deficiency; and 0.7% by other nutritional deficiencies.

As shown in Figure 3, out of the Int$ 39.82 billion fiscal value of NCD DALY lost in CEMAC, 9.3% were from malignant neoplasms (cancers); 0.4% from other neoplasms; 5.3% from diabetes mellitus; 5.8% from endocrine, blood, immune disorders; 10.4% from mental and substance use disorders; 4.6% from neurological conditions; 2.9% from sense organ diseases; 21.5% from cardiovascular diseases; 6.2% from respiratory diseases; 9.7% digestive diseases; 5.1% from genitourinary diseases; 1.9% from skin diseases; 4.4% musculoskeletal diseases; 11.4% from congenital anomalies; 0.8 from oral conditions; and 0.3% from sudden infant death syndrome.

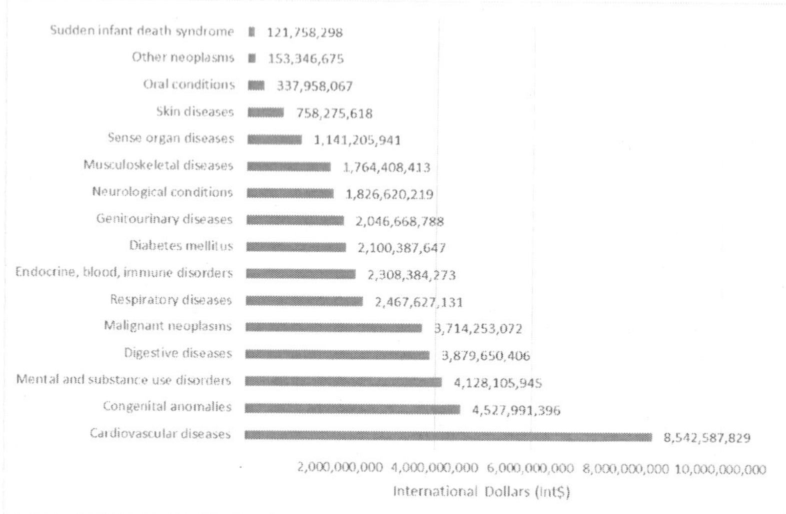

Source: Authors estimates.

Figure 3. Fiscal value of DALYs lost from non-communicable diseases in CEMAC (2015 Int$ or PPP).

Approximately 57.6% of the Int$ 3.7 billion fiscal value of DALYs lost from malignant neoplasms (cancer) was from mouth and oropharynx cancers, colon and rectum cancers, liver cancer, breast cancer, cervix uteri cancer, prostate cancer, and lymphomas or multiple myeloma.

Nearly 65% of the Int$4.1 billion fiscal value of mental and substance use disorders DALY losses were from depressive disorders, alcohol use disorders, drug use disorders, and anxiety disorders. About 74% of the Int$1.8 billion fiscal value of neurological conditions DALY losses were from epilepsy and migraine. Around 74% of the Int$1.1 billion fiscal value of sense organ diseases DALY losses were from uncorrected refractive errors, vision loss (excluding cataracts and glaucoma), and hearing loss.

Almost 70% of the Int$8.5 billion fiscal value of cardiovascular diseases DALY losses were from ischaemic heart disease and stroke. About 89% of the Int$2.5 billion fiscal value of respiratory diseases DALY losses were from asthma and chronic obstructive pulmonary disease. Nearly 69% of the Int$ 3.9 billion fiscal value of digestive diseases DALY losses were from peptic ulcer disease, cirrhosis of the liver, and paralytic ileus and intestinal obstruction. About 70% of the Int$ 2 billion fiscal value of genitourinary diseases DALY losses were from kidney and gynaecological diseases. Approximately 68% of the Int$ 1.8 billion fiscal value of musculoskeletal diseases DALY losses were from osteoarthritis, and back and neck pain. About 58% of the Int$ 4.5 billion fiscal value of congenital anomalies DALY losses were from neural tube defects and congenital heart anomalies. Nearby 60% of the Int$ 338 million fiscal value of oral conditions DALY losses were from edentulism and periodontal disease.

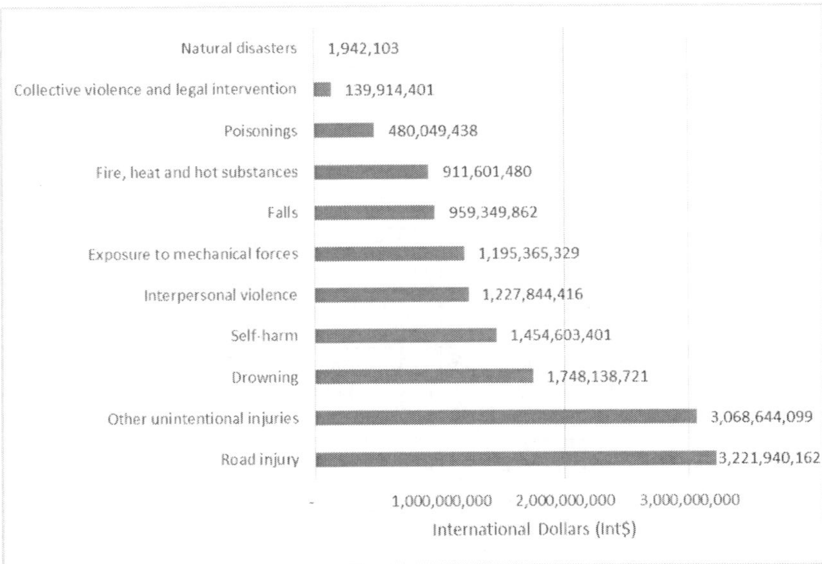

Source: Authors estimates.

Figure 4. Fiscal value of DALYs lost from injuries in CEMAC (2015 Int$ or PPP).

As portrayed in figure 4, out of the Int$ 14.41 billion fiscal value of injuries DALY lost in CEMAC, 80.4% was from unintentional (or accidental) injuries; and 19.6% was from intentional injuries.

Approximately 53% of the Int$ 11.6 billion fiscal value of DALYs lost from unintentional injuries was caused by road injuries, drowning and exposure to mechanical forces. Around 71% of the Int$ 2.8 billion fiscal value of DALYs lost from intentional injuries was attributed to self-harm and interpersonal violence. The financial values of DALYs lost from all the causes in CEMAC are contained in Appendix I.

Estimates of Reductions in Financial Values of DALY Losses in CEMAC Assuming the Five SDG 3 Related Targets Are Achieved

Table 4 presents the financial value of DALYs lost from SDG 3 health conditions in 2015 and 2030, and reductions in financial value of DALYs in 2030.

Table 4. CEMAC financial value of DALYs lost distributed by SDG health conditions

	(A). Financial Value of DALYS lost in 2015 (INT$)	Financial Value of DALYS lost in 2030 (INT$)	Reduction in Financial Value of DALYS lost in 2030 (INT$)
SDG 3.1: Maternal conditions	2,433,828,191	299,855,629	2,133,972,561
SDG 3.2: Neonatal conditions	17,444,662,680	7,152,709,071	10,291,953,608
SDG 3.3: Tuberculosis	2,757,693,366	275,769,337	2,481,924,029
SDG 3.3: HIV/AIDS	13,216,261,776	6,220,894,418	6,995,367,358
SDG 3.3: Malaria	6,733,757,084	673,375,708	6,060,381,376
SDG 3.3: NTDs (a+..+o)	2,329,135,591	582,283,898	1,746,851,693
(a). African Trypanosomiasis	151,260,667	37,815,167	113,445,500
(b). Schistosomiasis	601,233,773	150,308,443	450,925,330
(c). Leishmaniasis	2,672,425	668,106	2,004,319
(d). Lymphatic filariasis	201,169,271	50,292,318	150,876,953
(e). Onchocerciasis	399,011,958	99,752,989	299,258,968
(f). Cysticercosis	233,302,184	58,325,546	174,976,638
(g). Echinococcosis	6,072,180	1,518,045	4,554,135
(h). Dengue	18,032,957	4,508,239	13,524,718
(i). Trachoma	4,830,726	1,207,682	3,623,045
(j). Yellow fever	240,779,710	60,194,927	180,584,782
(k). Rabies	170,508,641	42,627,160	127,881,480
(l). Ascariasis	117,737,405	29,434,351	88,303,054
(m). Trichuriasis	40,194,121	10,048,530	30,145,591
(n). Hookworm disease	128,183,127	32,045,782	96,137,345

	(A). Financial Value of DALYS lost in 2015 (INT$)	**Financial Value of DALYS lost in 2030 (INT$)**	**Reduction in Financial Value of DALYS lost in 2030 (INT$)**
(o). Leprosy	14,146,447	3,536,612	10,609,835
SDG 3.4: Non-communicable diseases (a+..+p)	39,819,229,718	26,546,153,146	13,273,076,573
(a). Malignant neoplasms	3,714,253,072	2,476,168,715	1,238,084,357
(b). Other neoplasms	153,346,675	102,231,117	51,115,558
(c). Diabetes mellitus	2,100,387,647	1,400,258,431	700,129,216
(d). Endocrine, blood, immune disorders	2,308,384,273	1,538,922,849	769,461,424
(e). Mental and substance use disorders	4,128,105,945	2,752,070,630	1,376,035,315
(f). Neurological conditions	1,826,620,219	1,217,746,813	608,873,406
(g). Sense organ diseases	1,141,205,941	760,803,961	380,401,980
(h). Cardiovascular diseases	8,542,587,829	5,695,058,552	2,847,529,276
(i). Respiratory diseases	2,467,627,131	1,645,084,754	822,542,377
(j). Digestive diseases	3,879,650,406	2,586,433,604	1,293,216,802
(k). Genitourinary diseases	2,046,668,788	1,364,445,859	682,222,929
(l). Skin diseases	758,275,618	505,517,078	252,758,539
	(A). Financial Value of DALYS lost in 2015 (INT$)	Financial Value of DALYS lost in 2030 (INT$)	Reduction in Financial Value of DALYS lost in 2030 (INT$)
(m). Musculoskeletal diseases	1,764,408,413	1,176,272,276	588,136,138
(n). Congenital anomalies	4,527,991,396	3,018,660,931	1,509,330,465
(o). Oral conditions	337,958,067	225,305,378	112,652,689
(p). Sudden infant death syndrome	121,758,298	81,172,199	40,586,099
SDG 3.6: Road injury	3,221,940,162	1,610,970,081	1,610,970,081
TOTAL (INT$)	87,956,508,567	43,362,011,288	44,594,497,279

Source: Authors estimates.

The total financial value of DALYs lost from SDG 3 health conditions (maternal conditions, neonatal conditions, tuberculosis, HIV/AIDS, malaria, NTDs, NCDs and road injuries) in 2015 was Int$ 87,956,508,567. Whereas, the projected financial value of DALYs lost from the same SDG conditions in 2030 was Int$ 43,362,011,288. It is estimated that full attainment of SDG targets 3.1, 3.2, 3.3, 3.4 and 3.6 would save CEMAC Int$ 44,594,497,279.

DISCUSSION

The triple burden of communicable diseases, NCDs and injuries were responsible for loss of DALYs with a fiscal value of Int$140,106,558,107, which is approximately 59% of the sub-region's total GDP. The value of DALYs lost in CEMAC was lower than losses incurred by the AMU (12) and the EAC (14) of Int$ 289,033,271,814 and Int$ 203,843,476,166, respectively. As reported in the preceding section, CEMAC sub-region could potentially save Int$44,594,497,279 if SDG3 targets 3.1, 3.2, 3.3, 3.4 and 3.6 were fully achieved. For those targets to be fully achieved, the United Nations General Assembly (UNGA) political declarations and resolutions annotated below will need to be fully implemented by all six CEMAC member states.

SDG Target 3.1 and 3.2: Maternal, Neonatal and Child Health Conditions

Maternal Health

The CEMAC lost DALYs worth Int$ 2,433,828,191 in 2015 from maternal conditions. However, if SDG target 3.1 is fully achieved, the fiscal value of DALY losses in 2030 would be Int$ 299,855,629. This implies a saving of Int$ 2,133,972,561 per year.

The thirty-third session of UN Human Rights Council adopted resolution A/HRC/RES/33/18 entitled "Preventable maternal mortality and morbidity and human rights" (105). It recognizes preventing maternal mortality and morbidity as a human right. The resolution urges member states to implement a number of actions: assure women's universal access to quality maternity, sexual and reproductive health services, goods, information and education; integrate a human rights-based perspective into maternal mortality and morbidity initiatives; abolish discriminatory laws and combat gender stereotypes to ensure justice for women and girls; and strength maternal mortality and morbidity accountability mechanisms. It calls upon all Governments, national human rights institutions and civil society organizations, regional organizations, and relevant UN agencies, funds and programmes to support implementation of policies, strategies and interventions geared at achieving SDG target 3.1 of reducing the CEMAC maternal mortality ratio to less than 70 per 100,000 live births (99).

The twenty-second ordinary session of the Assembly of the African Union (AU) in January 2014 made a decision on progress on maternal new born and child health (MNCH) (106). The decision endorsed the recommendations contained in the 2013 status report on maternal, newborn and child health (107) and the action plan towards ending preventable maternal, newborn and child mortality (108).

The Twenty-Eighth Ordinary Session of the AU Assembly decided on universal access to immunization as a cornerstone for health and development in Africa (109). The decision calls upon Member States to allocate adequate domestic resources to strengthen national immunization programmes to achieve the Global Vaccine Action Plan goals; and to negotiate with vaccine manufacturers to ensure access to vaccines at affordable prices.

The Heads of State and Government of the AU at their 23rd Ordinary Session in June 2014 adopted a declaration on ending preventable child and maternal deaths in Africa (110). In that declaration they commit to end preventable child and maternal deaths by the year 2035; to develop and implement a Pan-African MNCH Road Map to facilitate achievement of universal access to quality MNCH services; and to support the development and adoption of a Pan-African MNCH Score Card to track progress (111, 112, 113).

Child Health

The CEMAC lost DALYs worth Int$ 17,444,662,680 in 2015 from neonatal conditions, including preterm birth complications, birth asphyxia and birth trauma, neonatal sepsis and infections. However, if SDG target 3.1 is fully achieved, the fiscal value of DALY losses in 2030 would be Int$ 7,152,709,071. This implies a saving of Int$ 10,291,953,608 per year. The SDG3 target 3.2 aspires to:

> "3.2 By 2030, end preventable deaths of newborns and children under 5 years of age, with all countries aiming to reduce neonatal mortality to at least as low as 12 per 1,000 live births and under-5 mortality to at least as low as 25 per 1,000 live births" (99).

In April 2013 the United Nations Human Right Council adopted resolution A/HRC/RES/22/32 entitled "Rights of the child: the right of the child to the enjoyment of the highest attainable standard of health" (114). The resolution calls upon states to ensure that the right of the child to the enjoyment of the highest attainable standard of physical and mental health promoted and protected through the enactment and implementation of laws, strategies and policies, gender- and child-responsive budgeting and resource allocation, and adequate investment in health systems; access to quality, affordable and equitable health care and social services; access to relevant information, education, counselling and services; universal free birth registration for all children; adopt a human rights-based approach to scale up integrated management of maternal, newborn and child health care; support national plans and programmes aimed at combating undernutrition in mothers and children; ensure a regular supply of safe and affordable drinking water and sanitation services of good quality; develop comprehensive policies and strategies to prevent harmful use of alcohol and illicit substances, and promote mental health during all stages of childhood; ensure sexual and reproductive health needs of children and adolescents are met, while assuring confidentiality and informed consent; prevent and to protect children from all forms of violence in all settings; ban all harmful practices compromising the dignity and integrity of the child; implement appropriate education, legislative, regulatory and fiscal measures to combat non-communicable disease risk factors, e.g., tobacco use, harmful use of alcohol, unhealthy diet and physical inactivity; providing care, support and treatment to children living with AIDS, their families and caregivers; develop multi-sectoral environmental health strategies to address the health conditions caused by environmental exposure to pollutants and other environmental harm; promote the full integration of palliative care services into treatment and support programmes for children with chronic illnesses; facilitate access to health services and medicines during emergencies; and build resilient and responsive health system to accelerate the transition towards universal health coverage.

In January 2018, the Seventy-second Session United Nations General Assembly (UNGA) adopted Resolution A/RES/72/154 entitled "The girl child" (115). The resolution, among others, urges States to improve the situation of girl children living in poverty, including extreme poverty, deprived of adequate food and nutrition, water and sanitation facilities, with limited or no access to basic physical and mental health-care services, shelter, education, participation and protection.

At Continent level, the AU Maputo plan of action 2016 – 2030, contains nine strategic areas of focus and priority interventions plus indicators for monitoring improvements maternal, newborn, child and adolescent health (111).

SDG Target 3.3: HIV/AIDs, Tuberculosis, Malaria and Neglected Tropical Diseases (NTD)

In 2015, the CEMAC lost DALYs valued at Int$ 13,216,261,776 from HIV/AIDS; Int$ 2,757,693,366 from tuberculosis; Int$ 6,733,757,084 from malaria; and Int$ 2,329,135,591 from NTD. If SDG 3.3 is achieved, the financial value of DALYs lost in 2030 from HIV/AIDS would be Int$ 6,220,894,418; from TB would be Int$ 275,769,337; from malaria would be Int$ 673,375,708; and from NTD would be Int$ 582,283,898. Thus, realization of SDG3.3 would save Int$ 6,995,367,358 from HIV/AIDS; Int$ 2,481,924,029 from TB; Int$ 6,060,381,376 from malaria; and Int$ 1,746,851,693 from reduced NTD burden. The CEMAC States might realize those savings if they fully implement their past commitments contained in the relevant UNGA Resolutions.

First, the UNGA committed to provide global, regional and sub-regional leadership, monitoring and accountability; increasing, diversifying and front-loading investments; ensure access to high-quality HIV services (including testing and treatment), commodities and prevention; contribute to gender equality and the empowerment of all women and girls; promoting laws, policies and practices to promote access and end HIV-related stigma and discrimination; and engage and support people living with HIV/AIDS to fast-track achievement of international targets aimed at ending AIDS epidemic by 2030 (116).

Second, on 5 October 2016 UNGA adopted a political declaration on antimicrobial resistance (AMR). It urges member states to develop adequately resourced multisectoral national action plans, programmes and policy initiatives to combat AMR; effective surveillance, monitoring and regulatory frameworks; awareness and knowledge-raising activities on AMR; and support a multisectoral One Health approach to tackle AMR (117).

Third, on 10 October 2018 UNGA adopted a political declaration underscoring need for urgent response to a global tuberculosis (TB) epidemic. It committed to develop/strengthen national TB strategic plans to implement rapidly the End TB Strategy and deliver the commitments contained in the UNGA TB political declaration; achieve effective universal access to quality diagnosis, treatment, care, and adherence support; legislating measures to prevent TB transmission in workplaces, schools, transportation systems, incarceration systems and other congregate settings; providing preventive treatment and other strategies; development of new TB vaccines; urgent response to multidrug-resistant TB; coordination and collaboration between TB and HIV programmes; integrating tuberculosis efforts fully into all relevant health services; developing community-based health services; improvements in related policies and public health systems; integrate digital technologies into existing health system infrastructures to enhance effectiveness of TB prevention, treatment and care; research and development of new tools for TB; pursue multisectoral collaboration at the global, regional, national and local levels; spearhead cooperation between public and private sector entities in development of medicines for multidrug-resistant and extensively drug-resistant TB; and mobilize adequate and sustainable financing for universal access to quality prevention, diagnosis, treatment and care of TB (118).

Fourth, on 10 September 2018 UNGA adopted resolution A/RES/72/309 that urges malaria-endemic countries to establish and/or strengthen national policies, operational plans and research; adopt a coordinated multisectoral approach to malaria control; increase the domestic resources for combatting the disease and to work towards financial sustainability; to effectively govern the recruitment, training, deployment and retention of skilled health personnel (including community health workers) to ensure availability of skilled personnel at all levels; strengthen health systems to ensure universal coverage of existing life-saving tools (including affordable quality medicines) for the prevention, diagnosis and treatment of malaria; continue to observe World Malaria Day on 25 April, in order to raise public awareness about the prevention and control of malaria; close collaboration with community leaders and implementing partners; and implement the Global Plan for Artemisinin Resistance Containment and the Global Plan for Insecticide Resistance Management in Malaria Vectors (119).

Finally, on 25 September 2015 UNGA adopted the 2030 Agenda containing 17 Sustainable Development Goals (SDGs) and 169 targets (99). The health SDG 3, target 3.3, aspires to end the epidemic neglected tropical diseases (NTDs) by 2030. The UN Commission on Population and Development Resolution E/CN.9/2010/9 urges member states to ensure prevention and treatment of NTDs (120). In the London declaration on NTDs, pharmaceutical companies, donors, endemic countries, and non-governmental organizations committed to extend and sustain drug access programmes; research and development into next-generation treatments; collaboration and coordination on NTDS at national and international levels; funding to implement NTD programmes; and monitoring and evaluation of NTD programmes (121).

SDG Target 3.4: Non-Communicable Diseases

In 2015, CEMAC lost NCD-related DALYs with a fiscal value of Int$ 39,819,229,718. If SDG target 3.4 on NCD is fully achieved, the financial value of DALYs lost in 2030 would be Int$ 26,546,153,146, which represents a saving of Int$ 13,273,076,573 per year. The CEMAC sub-regional economic community would stand a high probability of realizing that saving if member states implemented fully commitments contained in the UNGA resolutions on NCDs.

For instance, on 19 September 2011, sixty-sixth session of the UNGA adopted resolution A/RES/66/2 on prevention and control of NCDs, which called upon member states to develop and implement evidence-based multisectoral policies, programmes and action plans for prevention and control of NCD; accelerate implementation of the WHO Framework Convention on Tobacco Control (FCTC) to reduce availability and consumption of tobacco; accelerate implementation of the Global Strategy on Diet, Physical Activity and Health; implement the Global Strategy to Reduce the Harmful Use of Alcohol; legislate against production, marketing and sale of foods that contribute to unhealthy diet; implement cost-effective interventions to reduce salt, sugar and saturated fats; support exclusive breastfeeding for about six months from birth; increase access to cost-effective cancer screening services and vaccinations to prevent cancer; increase and prioritize budgetary allocations for addressing NCD risk factors; and strengthen all building blocks (pillars) of national health systems to efficiently and responsively deliver NCD services (122, 123).

On 10 October 2018 sixty-third session of UNGA adopted resolution A/RES/73/2 that called upon member states accelerate response to address NCDs for the health and well-being of present and future generations (124). It reaffirmed need to accelerate implementation of previous UNGA NCD-related resolutions (99, 122); provide strategic government leadership for the prevention and control of NCDs; implement own-country-led prioritized set of cost-effective, affordable and evidence-based NCD interventions and good practices; implement policy, legislative and regulatory measures to minimize impact of key risk factors and promote healthy diets and lifestyles; implement cost-effective interventions to halt the rise of overweight and obesity; establish or strengthen national multi-stakeholder dialogue mechanisms to fast-track implementation of national NCD prevention and control; scale up efforts to use information and communications technologies in prevention and control of NCD; and promote increased access to affordable, safe, effective and quality medicines and diagnostics and other technologies (124).

SDG Target 3.6: Road Traffic Injuries

In 2015, the CEMAC lost road injury-related DALYs with a fiscal value of Int$ 3,221,940,162. In its resolution 70/1 of 25 September 2015, entitled "Transforming our world: the 2030 Agenda for Sustainable Development," the UNGA set a SDG target 3.6 which aims to halve the number of global deaths and injuries from road traffic accidents by 2020 (99). Assuming CEMAC member states were to fully achieve SDG target 3.6, the fiscal value of DALYs lost from road injuries in 2030 would be Int$ 1,610,970,081, which signifies a saving of Int$ 1,610,970,081 per year.

The CEMAC sub-regional economic community might realize such a saving if member states were to implement fully the UNGA resolution A/RES/72/271 entitled "Improving global road safety" (125). That resolution recommends to member states to develop and implement national road safety plans; develop, enact and promulgate comprehensive legislation on key risk factors (non-use of seat belts, child restraints and helmets, drink-driving, and over speeding); enforce policies and measures to protect and promote pedestrian safety and cycling; proper planning and safety assessment, design, building and maintenance of roads; implement road safety management system; establish mechanisms for the periodic assessment of vehicles; implement appropriate social marketing campaigns to raise road safety awareness; implement professional driver qualification frameworks (training, certification and licensing); strengthen pre-hospital trauma care, hospital trauma care and rehabilitation services (125).

CONCLUSION

This study has estimated the fiscal value of DALYs lost in the CEMAC sub-region in 2015 without and with SDG 3. We have also reviewed briefly the recent SDG-related resolutions adopted by the UNGA, which if fully implemented could fast-track achievement of SDG 3 targets in CEMAC sub-region.

Were CEMAC to achieve the health SDG3 targets 3.1, 3.2, 3.3, 3.4 and 3.6 fully, the sub-region's total GDP would be expected to increase by at least 18.9%. Such economic dividends might be realized if CEMAC member states were to improve performance of their national and local health systems through an increase in health expenditures per capita to the level recommended for attainment of SDG3 (11). The reader should keep in mind the limitations of the human capital approach highlighted in literature review subsection.

Given the limitations of the human capital approach highlighted earlier, these kind of studies should be complemented with economic evaluation of alternative preventive, curative and rehabilitative interventions (126, 127) into diseases that result in the highest fiscal value of DALYs lost, to guide health policy development and decision-making in CEMAC member states.

ACKNOWLEDGMENTS

We owe profound gratitude to *Adonai Elohim* for inspiration and for meeting all our needs in the entire process of conceptualizing, analysing and writing this manuscript. The views expressed in this paper are those of authors only and should not be attributed to the African Sustainable Development Research Consortium (ASDRC).

References

[1] CEMAC. Les Etats membres de la CEMAC. URL https://www.cemac.int/.

[2] International Pecuniary Fund (IMF). World Economic Outlook Database, October 2015. Washington, DC, IMF. URL: http://www.imf.org/external/pubs/ft/weo/2015/02/weodata/weoselgr.aspx.

[3] World Health Organization (WHO). Global Health Estimates 2015: DALYs by Cause, Age, Sex, by Country and by Region, 2000-2015. Geneva: WHO, 2016.

[4] Sambo LG, Kirigia JM. Investing in health systems for universal health coverage in Africa. BMC Int Health Hum Rights 2014;14:28. URL: https://doi.org/10.1186/s12914-014-0028-5.

[5] Kirigia JM, Barry SP. Health challenges in Africa and the way forward. Int Arch Med 2008;1:27. URL: https://doi.org/10.1186/1755-7682-1-27.

[6] WHO. The World health report 2000 - health systems: improving performance. Geneva: WHO, 2000.

[7] Commission on Social Determinants of Health. Closing the gap in a generation: health equity through action on the social determinants of health: final report of the commission on social determinants of health. Geneva: WHO, 2008.

[8] Kirigia JM, Ota MO, Senkubuge F, Wiysonge CS, Mayosi BM. Developing the African national health research systems barometer. Health Res Policy Syst 2016; 14:53. URL: https://doi.org/10.1186/s12961-016-0121-4.

[9] WHO. World health statistics 2018: monitoring health for the SDGs, sustainable development goals. Geneva: WHO, 2018.

[10] WHO. World Health Statistics 2015. Geneva: WHO, 2015.

[11] Stenberg K, Hanssen O, Edejer TT, Bertram M, Brindley C, Meshreky A, et al. Financing transformative health systems towards achievement of the health sustainable development goals: A model for projected resource needs in 67 low-income and middle-income countries. Lancet Glob Health 2017;5:e875-87. URL: https://doi.org/10.1016/S2214-109X(17)30263-2.

[12] Muthuri RDK, Muthuri NG, Kirigia JM. Pecuniary value of disability-adjusted-life-years in the Arab Maghreb Union in 2015. J Hum Resource Sustain Stud 2018; 6:249-74.

[13] Acharya LD, Rau NR, Udupa N, Rajan MS, Vijayanarayana K. Assessment of cost of illness for diabetic patients in South Indian tertiary care hospital. J Pharm Bioallied Sci 2016;8(4):314–20.

[14] Kirigia JM, Mwabu GM. The monetary value of disability-adjusted-life-years lost in the East African Community in 2015. Modern Economy 2018;9:1360-77.

[15] Luengo-Fernande R, Leal J, Gray A, Sullivan R. Economic burden of cancer across the European Union: A population-based cost analysis. Lancet Oncol 2013;14:1165–74.

[16] Her Majesty the Queen in Right of Canada. Economic burden of illness in Canada, 2005–2008. Toronto: Public Health Agency Canada, 2014.

[17] Rice DP, Hodgson TA, Kopstein AN. The economic costs of illness: a replication and update. Health Care Financing Rev 1985;7(1):61-80.

[18] Laserna A, Barahona-Correa J, Baquero L, Castañeda-Cardona C, Rosselli D. Economic impact of dengue fever in Latin America and the Caribbean: a systematic review. Rev Panam Salud Publica 2018;42:e111. URL: https://doi.org/10.26633/RPSP.2018.111.

[19] Dupuit J. On the measurement of the utility of public works. In: Arrow K, Scitovsky T, eds. Readings in welfare economics. Homewood, IL: Irwin, 1969:255–83.

[20] Schelling TC. The life you save may be your own. In: Chase Jr SB, ed. Problems in public expenditure analysis. Washington, DC: Brookings Institute, 1968:127–62.

[21] Kirigia JM. The economics of schistosomiasis interventions: a cases study of the Mwea irrigation scheme in Kenya. Dissertation. York: University of York, 1994.

[22] Horowitz JK, McConnell KE. A review of WTP/WTA Studies. J Environ Econ Manag 2002;44:426–47.

[23] Kahneman D, Knetsch JL, Thaler RH. Experimental tests of the endowment effect and the Coase Theorem. Scott J Political Econ 1990;98(6):1325-48.

[24] Russel S, Fox-Rushby J, Arhin D. Willingness and ability to pay for health care: a selection of methods and issues. Health Policy Plan 1995;10(1):94-101.

[25] Simpkin AL, Schwartzstein RM. Tolerating uncertainty: The next medical revolution? N Engl J Med 2016;375(18):1714-5.

[26] Logan RL, Scott PJ. Uncertainty in clinical practice: implications for quality and costs of health care. Lancet 1996;347(9001):595-8.

[27] Jones-Lee MW. The value of life and safety: A survey of recent developments. Geneva Papers Risk Insurance 1985;10(36):141-73.

[28] Svensson M. The value of a statistical life in Sweden: Estimates from two studies using the "Certainty approach" calibration. Accid Anal Prev 2009;41(3):430-7.

[29] Haddak MM. Estimating the Willingness-to-pay for Road Safety Improvement. Transp Res A 2016; 14: 293-302. D.

[30] Andersson H. Willingness to pay for road safety and estimates of the risk of death: evidence from a Swedish contingent valuation study. Accid Anal Prev 2007;39(4): 853-65.

[31] Niroomanda N, Jenkins GP. Estimating the value of life and injury for pedestrians using a stated preference framework. J Safety Res 2017;62:81-7.

[32] Niroomanda N, Jenkins GP. Estimating the Value of Life, Injury, and Travel Time Saved Using a Stated Preference Framework. Accid Anal Prev 2016;91:216-25.

[33] Diener A, O'Brien B, Gafni A. Health care contingent valuation studies: A review and classification of the literature. Health Econ 1998;7:313-26.

[34] Latif E. Monetary valuation of cardiovascular disease in Canada. Econ Bus Lett 2012; 1(1):46-52.

[35] Krupnick A, Alberini A, Cropper M, Simon N, O'Brien B, Goeree R, Heintzelman M. Age, Health and the willingness to pay for mortality risk reductions: A contingent valuation survey of Ontario residents. J Risk Uncertain 2002;24(2):161–86.

[36] Jofre-Bonet M, Kamara J. Willingness to pay for health insurance in the informal sector of Sierra Leone. PLoS One 2018;13(5):e0189915. URL: https://doi.org/10.1371/journal.pone.0189915.

[37] Dong H, Kouyate B, Cairns J, Mugisha F, Sauerborn R. (2003) Willingness-to-pay for community-based insurance in Burkina Faso. Health Econ 2003;12(10) 849–62.

[38] Donfouet HPP, Makaudze E, Mahieu P-A, Malin E. The determinants of the willingness-to-pay for com- munity-based prepayment scheme in rural Cameroon. Int J Health Care Finance Econ 2011;11(3):209–20.

[39] Asfaw A, von Braun J. Can community health insurance schemes shield the poor against the downside health effects of economic reforms? The case of rural Ethiopia. Health policy 2004;70(1):97–108.

[40] Asenso-Okyere WK, Osei-Akoto I, Anum A, Appiah EN. (1997) Willingness to pay for health insurance in a developing economy. A pilot study of the informal sector of Ghana using contingent valuation. Health Policy 1997;42(3):223–37.

[41] Oyibo PG, Ejughemre UJ. Willingness to pay for community health insurance in a semi-urban community in Delta State, Nigeria. Highland Med Res J 2015;15(2):83-7.

[42] Onwujekwe O, Okereke E, Onoka C, Uzochukwu B, Kirigia J, Petu A. (2009). Willingness to pay for community-based health insurance in Nigeria: Do economic status and place of residence matter? Health Policy Plan 2009; 25(2): 155–61.

[43] Oyekale AS. Factors influencing Households' willingness to pay for National Health Insurance Scheme (NHIS) in Osun state, Nigeria. Stud Ethno-Med 2012;6(3):167–72.

[44] Omotowo IB, Ezeoke UE, Obi IE, Uzochukwu BSC, Agunwa CC, Eke CB, et al. Household perceptions, willingness to pay, benefit package preferences, health system readiness for National Health Insurance scheme in Southern Nigeria. Health 2016;8: 1630-44.

[45] Basaza R, Alier PK, Kirabira P, Ogubi D, Lako RLL. Willingness to pay for National Health Insurance Fund among public servants in Juba City, South Sudan: A contingent evaluation. Int J Equity Health 2017;16:158.

[46] Damali D, Robert A, Onzima RADDM, Philip G, Katongole S, Ayiko R, Nabyonga-Orem J. Communities' willingness to pay for healthcare in public health facilities of Nakasongola District, Uganda. Int J Public Health Res 2015;3(5):248-53.

[47] Masiye F, Rehnberg C. The economic value of an improved malaria treatment programme in Zambia: results from a contingent valuation survey. Malar J 2005; 4:60.

[48] Paulo EC, Forsberg BC, Premji Z, Montogomery SM, Bjorkman A. Willingness and ability to pay for artemisinin-based combination therapy in rural Tanzania. Malar J 2008;7:227.

[49] Adeneye AK, Mafe MA, Appelt B, Idowu ET, Akande DO. Willingness to pay for praziquantel treatment in a hyperendemic community of Ogun State, Nigeria. Res Social Adm Pharm 2006;2(1):83-95.

[50] Ramakrishnan G, Tuchman J, Hartel J. Willingness to pay for condoms in five countries: Kenya, Nigeria, South Africa, Zambia, and Zimbabwe. Arlington, VA: Strengthening High Impact Interventions for an AIDS-free Generation (AIDSFree) Project, 2018.

[51] Ternent L, McNamee P, Newlands D, Belemsaga D, Gbangou A, Cross S. Willingness to pay for maternal health outcomes: Are women willing to pay more than men? Appl Health Econ Health Policy 2010;8(2):99–109.

[52] Kirigia JM, Sambo LG, Kainyu LH. Willingness-to-pay for schistosomiasis-related health outcomes in Kenya. Afr J Health Sci 2000;7(3-4):55-67.

[53] Acton JP. Measuring the monetary value of life saving programmes. Law Contemp Probl 1976;40(4):46-72.

[54] Hicks J. The foundations of welfare economics. Econ J 1939;49(196):696–712.

[55] Kaldor N. Welfare propositions in economics and interpersonal comparisons of utility. Econ J 1939;49(195):549–52.

[56] Gafni A. Willingness to pay in the context of an economic evaluation of healthcare programmes: theory and practice. Am J Manag Care 1997;3(Suppl):S21-S32.

[57] Gafni A. Using willingness-to-pay as a measure of benefits: what is the relevant question to ask in the context of public decision-making about health care programmes? Med Care 1991;29:1246-52.

[58] Fishchoff B, Cox LA. Conceptual framework for regulatory benefits assessment, In: Bentkover lD, Covella VT, Mumpower J, eds. Benefits assessment: The state of the art. Boston: MA: D Reidel Publishing Company, 1986.

[59] Payne SL. The art of asking questions. Princeton, NJ: Princeton University Press, 1952.

[60] Cookson R. Willingness-to-pay methods in healthcare: A sceptical view. Health Econ 2003;12(11):891–4.

[61] Kahneman D, Knetsch JL. Valuing public goods: the purchase of moral satisfaction. J Environ Econ Manag 1992;22(1):57-70.

[62] Smith RD, Sach TH. Contingent valuation: what needs to be done? Health Econ Policy Law 2010;5:91-111.

[63] Organisation for Economic Co-Operation and Development (OECD). The well-being of nations: The role of human and social capital. Paris: OECD, 2001.

[64] Lundvall B, Johnson B. The learning economy. J Industry Stud 1994;1(2):23-42.

[65] Murray CJL. Quantifying the burden of disease: The technical basis for disability-adjusted life years. Bull World Health Organ 1994;72(3):429-45.

[66] Weisbrod BA. The valuation of human capital. J Political Econ 1961;69(5):425-36.

[67] Robinson LA, Hammitt JK. Valuing reductions in fatal illness risks: Implications of recent research. Health Econ 2016;25(8):1039-52.

[68] Hurd MD, Martorell P, Delavande A, Mullen KJ, Langa KM. Monetary Costs of Dementia in the United States. N Engl J Med 2013;368(14):1326-34.

[69] DeVol R, Bedroussian A. An unhealthy America: The economic burden of chronic disease charting a new course to save lives and increase productivity and economic growth. Santa Monica, CA: Milken Institute, 2007.

[70] Castaneda-Orjuela C, Dıaz H, Alvis-Guzman N, Olarte A, Rodriguez H, Camargo G, et al. Burden of disease and economic impact of dengue and severe dengue in Colombia, 2011. Value Health Reg Issues 2012; 1(2): 123–128.

[71] Bloom DE, Chen S, McGovern ME. The economic burden of noncommunicable diseases and mental health conditions: Results for Costa Rica, Jamaica, and Peru. Rev Panam Salud Publica 2018;42:e18.

[72] Olesen J, Gustavsson A, Svensson M, Wittchen H-U, Jonsson B. The economic cost of brain disorders in Europe. The economic cost of brain disorders in Europe. Eur J Neurol 2012;19:155–62.

[73] Luengo-Fernandez R, Leal J, Gray A, Petersen S, Rayner M. Cost of cardiovascular diseases in the United Kingdom. Heart 2006;92(10):1384–9.

[74] Liu, JLY, Maniadakis N, Gray A, Rayner M. The economic burden of coronary heart disease in the UK. Heart 2002;88(6):597–603.

[75] Collins D, Hafidz F, Mustikawati D. The economic burden of tuberculosis in Indonesia Int J Tuberc Lung Dis 2017;21(9):1041-8.

[76] Pitayatienanan P, Butchon R, Yothasamut J, Aekplakorn W, Teerawattananon Y, Suksomboon N, et al. Economic costs of obesity in Thailand: a retrospective cost-of-illness study. BMC Health Serv Res 2014;14:146.

[77] Ranaweera S, Amarasinghe H, Chandraratne N, Thavorncharoensap M, Ranasinghe T, Karunaratna S, et al. Economic costs of alcohol use in Sri Lanka. PLoS One 2018; 13(6):e0198640.

[78] Amarasinghe H, Ranaweera S, Ranasinghe T, Chandraratne N, Kumara DR, Thavorncharoensap M, et al. Economic cost of tobacco-related cancers in Sri Lanka. Tob Control 2018;27:542–6.

[79] Xu J, Wang J, Wimo A, Fratiglioni L, Qiu C. The economic burden of dementia in China, 1990–2030: implications for health policy. Bull World Health Organ 2017;95: 18-26.

[80] Hayata E, Seto K, Haga K, Kitazawa T, Matsumoto K, Morita M, Hasegawa T. Cost of illness of the Cervical Cancer of the uterus in Japan - a time trend and future projections. BMC Health Serv Res 2015;15:104. URL: https://doi.org/10.1186/s12913-015-0776-5.

[81] Peabody JW, Shimkhada R, Tan C, Luck J. The burden of disease, economic costs and clinical consequences of tuberculosis in the Philippines. Health Policy Plann 2005;20(6):347-53.

[82] Kirigia JM, Mwabu MG, M'Imunya JM, Muthuri RDK, Nkanata LHK, Gitonga EB. Indirect Cost of Non-Communicable Diseases Deaths in the World Health Organization African Region. Int Arch Med 2017;10(34):1-21. URL: https://doi.org/10.3823/2304.

[83] Kirigia JM, Mburugu GN. The monetary value of human lives lost due to neglected tropical diseases in Africa. Infect Dis Poverty 2017;6:165. URL: https://doi.org/10.1186/s40249-017-0379-y.

[84] Cook PJ. The value of human life in the demand for safety: comment. Am Econ Rev 1978;68(4):710-1.

[85] Viscusi Labour market valuations of life and limb: empirical evidence and policy implications. Public Policy 1978;26(3):359-86.

[86] Jones-Lee MW. The economics of safety and physical risk. Oxford: Basil Blackwell, 1989.

[87] Mishan EJ. Cost-Benefit Analysis. London: Unwin Hyman, 1971.

[88] Mooney GH. The valuation of human life. London: Macmillan, 1977.

[89] Culyer AJ, Simpson H. Externality models and health: A Rückblick over the last twenty years. Econ Record 1980;56(154) 222-30.

[90] Margolis H. Selfishness, altruism and rationality. Cambridge: Cambridge University Press, 1982.

[91] Muthuri RNDK. Predictors of altruistic behavior among sample of emerging adults at the United States International University in Africa. Ann Behav Sci 2018;4(2):4. doi: 10.21767/2471-7975.100035.

[92] McGuire A, Henderson J, Mooney G. The economics of health care. London: Routledge Kegan Paul, 1988.

[93] Acton JP. Demand for health care when time prices vary more than money prices. Paper No. R-1189OEO/NYC, 973. Santa Monica, CA: Rand Corporation, 1973.

[94] Robinson JC. Philosophical Origins of the Economic Valuation of Life. Milbank Q 1986;64(1) 133-55.

[95] Mooney G, Creese A. Priority setting for health services efficiency: the role of measurement of burden of illness. In: Jamison DT, Mosley WH, Meashem AR, Bobadilla JL, eds. Disease control priorities in developing countries. New York: Oxford University Press, 1993.

[96] Shiell A, Gerald K, Donaldson C. Cost of illness studies: An aid to decision-making? Health Policy 1987;8:317-23.

[97] Kirigia JM, Mburugu GN, Huka GS. The indirect cost of disability adjusted life years lost among the elderly in Kenya. Int Arch Med 2017;10(213):1-14. URL: https://doi.org/10.3823/2483.

[98] WHO. WHO guide to identifying the economic consequences of disease and injury. Geneva: WHO, 2009.

[99] United Nations (UN). Transforming our world: the 2030 Agenda for Sustainable Development. Seventieth session of the United Nations General Assembly Resolution A/RES/70/1. New York: UN, 2015.

[100] WHO. Global Health Sector Strategy on HIV 2016-2021: Towards Ending AIDS. The Sixty-Ninth World Health Assembly Document A69/31. Geneva: WHO, 2016.

[101] WHO. Global technical strategy for malaria 2016-2030. Geneva: WHO, 2015.

[102] WHO. The end TB strategy. Geneva: WHO, 2015.

[103] WHO. Global vector control response 2017–2030. Geneva: WHO, 2017.

[104] WHO. Global Health Expenditure Database. Geneva: WHO, 2017. URL: http://apps.who.int/nha/database/Select/Indicators/en.

[105] UN. Preventable maternal mortality and morbidity and human rights. Human Rights Council Resolution A/HRC/RES/33/18. New York: UN, 2018.

[106] African Union (AU). Decision on Progress on Maternal, New Born and Child Health (MNCH). AU Assembly Decision Assembly/AU/Dec.494(XXII). Addis Ababa: AU, 2014.

[107] AU. 2013 Status Report on Maternal, Newborn & Child Health. Addis Ababa: AU, 2013.

[108] AU. 1st African Union International Conference on Maternal, Newborn and Child Health: Plan of Action Towards Ending Preventable Maternal, Newborn and Child Mortality. Addis Ababa: AU, 2013.

[109] AU. Decision on universal access to immunization as a cornerstone for health and development in Africa. Doc. EX.CL/1002(XXX)Add.1. Twenty-Eighth Ordinary Session of the African Union Assembly decision Assembly/AU/Dec.624(XXVIII). Addis Ababa: AU, 2017.

[110] AU. Declaration on Ending Preventable Child and Maternal Death in Africa – Doc. Assembly/AU/18(XXIII) Add.3. Declaration Assembly/AU/Decl.2(XXIII). Addis Ababa: AU, 2014.

[111] AU. Maputo plan of action 2016 – 2030 for the operationalisation of the continental policy framework for sexual and reproductive health and rights. Addis Ababa: AU, 2016.

[112] UN. Eliminating preventable maternal mortality and morbidity through the empowerment of women. Commission on the Status of Women Resolution E/CN.6/2010/L.6. New York: UN, 2010.

[113] African Union (AU) Maputo plan of action 2016 – 2030 for the operationalisation of the continental policy framework for sexual and reproductive health and rights. Addis Ababa: AU, 2016.

[114] UN. Rights of the child: the right of the child to the enjoyment of the highest attainable standard of health. Human Right Council Resolution A/HRC/RES/22/32. Geneva: UN, 2013.

[115] UN. The girl child. Seventy-second session General Assembly Resolution A/RES/72/154. New York: UN, 2018.

[116] UN. Political Declaration on HIV and AIDS: On the Fast Track to Accelerating the Fight against HIV and to Ending the AIDS Epidemic by 2030. UN General Assembly Resolution A/RES/70/266. New York: UN, 2016.

[117] UN. Political declaration of the high-level meeting of the General Assembly on antimicrobial resistance. Resolution A/RES/71/3. New York: UN, 2016.

[118] UN. Political declaration of the high-level meeting of the General Assembly on the fight against tuberculosis. United to end tuberculosis: An urgent global response to a global epidemic. UNGA Resolution A/RES/73/3. New York: UN, 2018.

[119] UN. Consolidating gains and accelerating efforts to control and eliminate malaria in developing countries, particularly in Africa, by 2030. UNGA Resolution A/RES/72/309. New York: UN, 2018.

[120] UN. Health, morbidity, mortality and development. Commission on Population and Development Resolution 2010/1. New York: UN, 2010.

[121] Uniting to Combat NTDs. London declaration on neglected tropical diseases. Ending the neglect and reaching 2020 goals. London: Uniting to Combat NTDs, 2012.

[122] UN. Political Declaration of the High-level Meeting of the General Assembly on the Prevention and Control of Non-communicable Diseases. Resolution A/RES/66/2. New York: UN, 2011.

[123] UN. Outcome document of the high-level meeting of the General Assembly on the comprehensive review and assessment of the progress achieved in the prevention and control of non-communicable diseases. Resolution A/RES/68/300. New York: UN, 2014.

[124] UN. Political declaration of the third high-level meeting of the General Assembly on the prevention and control of non-communicable diseases. UNGA Resolution A/RES/73/2. New York: UN, 2018.

[125] UN. Improving global road safety. Resolution A/RES/72/271. New York: UN, 2018.

[126] Kirigia JM. Economic evaluation of public health problems in sub-Saharan Africa. Nairobi: University of Nairobi Press, 2009.

[127] Drummond MF, Sculpher MJ, Torrance GW, O'Brien BJ, Stoddart GL. Methods for the Economic Evaluation of Health Care Programmes. London: Oxford University Press, 2005.

APPENDIX I. CEMAC FINANCIAL VALUE OF DALYS LOST DISTRIBUTED BY DISEASES

Diseases/Health Conditions	**Financial Value of DALYs lost (2015 Int$ or PPP)***
All Causes (I+II+III)	140,106,558,107
(I) Communicable, maternal, perinatal and nutritional conditions (A+B+C+D+E)	*85,877,934,976*
(A) *Infectious and parasitic diseases (1+2+3+...+12)*	45,119,363,969
1) Tuberculosis	2,757,693,366
2) STDs excluding HIV *(a+b+c+d+e+f)*	1,378,440,120
a) Syphilis	1,267,526,423
b) Chlamydia	29,825,039
c) Gonorrhoea	49,988,905
d) Trichomoniasis	8,426,479
e) Genital herpes	7,882,832
f) Other STDs	14,790,442
3) HIV/AIDS	13,216,261,776
4) Diarrhoeal diseases	9,402,566,565
5) Childhood-cluster diseases (a+b+c+d)	3,021,175,324
a) Whooping cough	800,966,114
b) Diphtheria	71,866,854
c) Measles	1,693,471,884
d) Tetanus	454,870,471
6) Meningitis	3,572,274,068
7) Encephalitis	227,818,134
8) Hepatitis	322,359,408
a) Acute hepatitis A	53,086,921
b) Acute hepatitis B	139,199,244
c) Acute hepatitis C	8,953,716
d) Acute hepatitis E	121,119,527
9) Parasitic and vector diseases (a+b+c+…+m)	8,762,631,576
a) Malaria	6,733,757,084
b) African Trypanosomiasis	151,260,667
c) Chagas disease	-
d) Schistosomiasis	601,233,773
e) Leishmaniasis	2,672,425
f) lymphatic filariasis	201,169,271
g) Onchocerciasis	399,011,958
h) Cysticercosis	233,302,184
i) Echinococcosis	6,072,180
j) Dengue	18,032,957
k) Trachoma	4,830,726

Appendix I. (Continued)

Diseases/Health Conditions	Financial Value of DALYs lost (2015 Int$ or PPP)*
l) Yellow fever	240,779,710
m) Rabies	170,508,641
10) Intestinal nematode infections (a+b+c+d)	286,114,652
a) Ascariasis	117,737,405
b) Trichuriasis	40,194,121
c) Hookworm disease	128,183,127
d) Food-bourne trematodes	-
11) Leprosy	14,146,447
12) Other infectious diseases	2,157,882,534
(B) Respiratory Infectious (1+2+3)	15,176,122,483
1) Lower respiratory infections	14,915,507,993
2) Upper respiratory infections	104,513,404
3) Otitis media	156,101,086
C) Maternal conditions	2,433,828,191
D) Neonatal conditions	17,444,662,680
1) Preterm birth complications	6,846,107,567
2) Birth asphyxia and birth trauma	6,564,933,338
3) Neonatal sepsis and infections	2,987,139,070
4) Other neonatal conditions	1,046,482,704
E) Nutritional deficiencies (1+2+3+4+5)	5,703,957,654
1) Protein-energy malnutrition	3,207,461,510
2) Iodine deficiency	101,448,289
3) Vitamin A deficiency	13,464,769
4) Iron-deficiency anaemia	2,342,516,513
5) Other nutritional deficiencies	39,066,574
(II) Noncommunicable diseases	*39,819,229,718*
(A) Malignant neoplasms	3,714,253,072
1) Mouth and oropharynx cancers (a+b+c)	209,400,499
a) Lip and oral cavity	77,187,178
b) Nasopharynx	50,432,076
c) Other pharynx	81,781,245
2) Oesophagus cancer	66,113,385
3) Stomach cancer	104,527,997
4) Colon and rectum cancers	175,701,730
5) Liver cancer (a+b+c+d)	329,254,889
a) Liver cancer secondary to hepatitis B	164,885,436
b) Liver cancer secondary to hepatitis C	47,996,116
c) Liver cancer secondary to alcohol use	90,819,940
d) Other liver cancer	25,553,397
6) Pancreas cancer	36,536,057

Diseases/Health Conditions	**Financial Value of DALYs lost (2015 Int$ or PPP)***
7) Trachea, bronchus, lung cancers	107,324,567
8) Melanoma and other skin cancers (a+b)	37,736,741
a) Malignant skin melanoma	24,779,813
b) Non-melanoma skin cancer	12,956,929
9) Breast cancer	462,624,587
10) Cervix uteri cancer	325,498,629
11) Corpus uteri cancer	33,132,746
12) Ovary cancer	101,198,054
13) Prostate cancer	167,515,184
14) Testicular cancer	6,361,873
15) Kidney cancer	67,344,405
16) Bladder cancer	37,228,149
17) Brain and nervous system cancers	51,460,056
18) Gallbladder and biliary tract cancer	4,449,652
19) Larynx cancer	22,874,321
20) Thyroid cancer	12,323,998
21) Mesothelioma (a+b+c)	71,704
22) Lymphomas, multiple myeloma	469,288,331
a) Hodgkin lymphoma	29,821,706
b) Non-Hodgkin lymphoma	415,898,625
c) Multiple myeloma	23,568,000
22) Leukaemia	133,614,917
24) Other malignant neoplasms	752,670,600
(B) Other neoplasms	153,346,675
(C) Diabetes mellitus	2,100,387,647
(D) Endocrine, blood, immune disorders (1+2+3+4)	2,308,384,273
1) Thalassaemias	51,798,205
2) Sickle cell disorders and trait	1,541,548,336
3) Other haemoglobinopathies and haemolytic anaemias	235,947,030
4) Other endocrine, blood and immune disorders	479,090,702
E) Mental and substance use disorders	4,128,105,945
1) Depressive disorders (a+b)	1,438,020,019
a) Major depressive disorder	1,224,696,722
b) Dysthymia	213,323,298
2) Bipolar disorder	214,321,380
3) Schizophrenia	243,276,574
4) Alcohol use disorders	311,565,779
5) Drug use disorders (a+b+c+d+e)	412,274,034
a) Opioid use disorders	382,531,620
b) Cocaine use disorders	6,239,821
c) Amphetamine use disorders	4,802,078
d) Cannabis use disorders	8,319,152
e) Other drug use disorders	10,381,363

Appendix I. (Continued)

Diseases/Health Conditions	**Financial Value of DALYs lost (2015 Int$ or PPP)***
6) Anxiety disorders	518,074,540
7) Eating disorders	30,868,660
8) Autism and Asperger syndrome	283,807,562
9) Childhood behavioural disorders (a+b)	257,509,422
a) Attention deficit/hyperactivity syndrome	18,489,733
b) Conduct disorder	239,019,689
10) Idiopathic intellectual disability	219,722,016
11) Other mental and behavioural disorders	198,665,959
(F) Neurological conditions (1+2+3+4+5+6+7)	1,826,620,219
1) Alzheimer disease and other dementias	259,740,928
2) Parkinson disease	20,848,817
3) Epilepsy	822,705,805
4) Multiple sclerosis	8,041,068
5) Migraine	529,320,277
6) Non-migraine headache	68,964,487
7) Other neurological conditions	116,998,836
(G) Sense organ diseases (1+2+3+4+5+6+7)	1,141,205,941
1) Glaucoma	20,563,811
2) Cataracts	125,752,356
3) Uncorrected refractive errors	179,235,447
4) Macular degeneration	31,183,260
5) Other vision loss	171,375,322
6) Other hearing loss	493,657,242
7) Other sense organ disorders	119,438,504
(H) Cardiovascular diseases	8,542,587,829
1) Rheumatic heart disease	326,104,547
2) Hypertensive heart disease	519,153,148
3) Ischaemic heart disease	2,647,216,941
4) Stroke	3,305,054,156
a) Ischaemic stroke	969,262,441
b) Haemorrhagic stroke	2,335,791,715
5) Cardiomyopathy, myocarditis, endocarditis	461,138,197
6) Other circulatory diseases	1,283,920,840
(I) Respiratory diseases (1+2+3)	2,467,627,131
1) Chronic obstructive pulmonary disease	847,199,863
2) Asthma	1,346,271,896
3) Other respiratory diseases	274,155,373
(J) Digestive diseases	3,879,650,406
1) Peptic ulcer disease	380,243,307
2) Cirrhosis of the liver (a+b+c+d)	1,907,300,226

Diseases/Health Conditions	**Financial Value of DALYs lost (2015 Int$ or PPP)***
a) Cirrhosis due to hepatitis B	602,559,733
b) Cirrhosis due to hepatitis C	217,085,194
c) Cirrhosis due to alcohol use	722,666,259
d) Other liver cirrhosis	364,989,039
3) Appendicitis	188,827,328
4) Gastritis and duodenitis	227,309,623
5) Paralytic ileus and intestinal obstruction	404,208,550
6) Inflammatory bowel disease	108,931,528
7) Gallbladder and biliary diseases	161,550,140
8) Pancreatitis	137,316,650
9) Other digestive diseases	363,963,053
(K) Genitourinary diseases	2,046,668,788
1) Kidney diseases (a+b+c)	1,197,348,280
a) Acute glomerulonephritis	3,628,392
b) Chronic kidney disease due to diabetes	229,686,944
c) Other chronic kidney disease	964,032,945
2) Benign prostatic hyperplasia	31,405,534
3) Urolithiasis	8,200,711
4) Other urinary diseases	436,554,799
5) Infertility	128,383,756
6) Gynecological diseases	244,775,708
(L) Skin diseases	758,275,618
(M) Musculoskeletal diseases (1+2+3+4+5)	1,764,408,413
1) Rheumatoid arthritis	101,419,028
2) Osteoarthritis	193,026,361
3) Gout	20,769,199
4) Back and neck pain	1,014,168,150
5) Other musculoskeletal disorders	435,025,676
(N) Congenital anomalies (1+2+3+4+5+6)	4,527,991,396
1) Neural tube defects	849,585,445
2) Cleft lip and cleft palate	2,504,525
3) Down syndrome	147,021,196
4) Congenital heart anomalies	1,757,109,440
5) Other chromosomal anomalies	256,411,925
6) Other congenital anomalies	1,515,358,865
(O) Oral conditions	337,958,067
1) Dental caries	43,645,801
2) Periodontal disease	85,544,050
3) Edentulism	118,368,017
4) Other oral disorders	90,400,200
(P) Sudden infant death syndrome	121,758,298
(III) Injuries	*14,409,393,413*

Appendix I. (Continued)

Diseases/Health Conditions	**Financial Value of DALYs lost (2015 Int$ or PPP)***
(A) Unintentional injuries (1+2+3+4+5+6+7+8)	11,587,031,195
1) Road injury	3,221,940,162
2) Poisonings	480,049,438
3) Falls	959,349,862
4) Fire, heat and hot substances	911,601,480
5) Drowning	1,748,138,721
6) Exposure to mechanical forces	1,195,365,329
7) Natural disasters	1,942,103
8) Other unintentional injuries	3,068,644,099
(B) Intentional injuries (1+2+3)	2,822,362,219
1) Self-harm	1,454,603,401
2) Interpersonal violence	1,227,844,416
3) Collective violence and legal intervention	139,914,401

Source: *Fiscal value of DALYs lost (2015 Int$ or PPP) are authors estimates.

In: Disability: International Aspects
Editors: Ariel Tenenbaum et al.
ISBN: 978-1-53617-886-9

Chapter 6

SHIFTING SANDS? ASSESSING THE SOCIAL INCLUSION OF PERSONS WITH DISABILITIES IN ALGIERS

Paula C Pinto*, PhD, Teresa J Pinto, PhD Candidate and Albino Cunha, PhD

Disability and Human Rights Observatory, Center for Interdisciplinary Gender Studies, Center for Administration and Public Policy, School of Social and Political Sciences (ISCSP), University of Lisbon, Lisbon, Portugal

ABSTRACT

Social inclusion of persons with disabilities has become a pressing issue in Algeria, particularly following the country's ratification of the Convention on the Rights of Persons with Disabilities (CRPD) in 2009. This paper presents the results of a study that aimed to understand the factors that hinder or facilitate the social inclusion of persons with

* Corresponding Author: Associate Professor Paula Campos Pinto, Disability and Human Rights Observatory, CIEG/ISCSP, University of Lisbon, Rua Almerindo Lessa, 1300-663 Lisbon, Portugal. E-mail: ppinto@iscsp.ulisboa.pt.

disabilities in the region of Algiers. The study uses a mixed-methods approach that included a questionnaire (n=285) and semi-structured interviews (n=48) applied to persons with disabilities aged 15-45 years in Algiers. Results showed that despite the growing recognition of persons with disabilities rights within the Algerian legal and policy framework, important gaps persist in the implementation of those rights. An extreme economic vulnerability, low educational levels and obstacles to inclusion in the labour market are still evident. Lack of physical accessibility, discrimination against persons with disabilities in the labour market and the persistence of negative attitudes towards persons with disabilities in public services and in society in general (e.g., labelling; staring; lack of respect for priority) are further obstacles reported. This chapter discusses the implication of these results for Algeria's compliance with the norms and principles of the CRPD.

INTRODUCTION

Over the past few decades, Algeria has made significant progress in the development of policy to support the social inclusion of its citizens with disabilities. In particular through the adoption of Law 02-09, which regulates the Protection and Promotion of the Rights of People with Disabilities, the Algerian State has developed new provisions to advance the social participation, education, vocational training, employment, health and rehabilitation of its disabled citizens. This national commitment was reinforced by the ratification of the UN Convention on the Rights of Persons with Disabilities (CRPD) in 2009. In this international Convention, social inclusion is described as a general principle (article 3), an obligation of Member-States (article 4) and a right of persons with disabilities (see for example articles 19, 29 and 30), thus emphasizing that participation plays a crucial role to the fulfillment of the rights-based paradigm proposed by the CRPD.

Nonetheless, reports from civil society organizations (1, 2) raise concerns about the efficacy of these new measures and suggest that persons with disabilities continue to be a disenfranchised and largely excluded group in the country, as it is also the case in other states of the African continent (3, 4). It thus becomes relevant to investigate the factors that hinder and facilitate the social inclusion of persons with disabilities in the region. Drawing from 285 questionnaires and 48 interviews conducted with persons disabilities, aged 15-45 years old living in the capital city of Algiers, this paper sets out to examine this question, and discuss its human rights implications.

Understanding disability and social inclusion

Disability is a highly complex and evolving notion. Since at least the late 1970s, the so-called social model of disability has been questioning prevailing biomedical understandings of disability, asserting that individual impairments do not imply, by themselves, a social disadvantage, since it is society, rather than biology, that disables some individuals (5-7). A new aim for social policy has thus been identified – the elimination of barriers that prevent equal participation (8).

This shift from an individual to a sociocultural understanding of disability had profound political, economic and social effects and strengthened the political expression of the disability movement worldwide (9, 10). Supported by this increasingly international movement, important steps to promote the rights of persons with disabilities were taken, culminating in the enactment of the Convention on the Rights of Persons with Disabilities (CRPD) by the United Nations Assembly in 2006.

The CRPD frames disability as a human rights issue and asserts the rights of all disabled people to equal citizenship. Advancing an understanding of disability that recognizes the interaction between personal, social and environmental factors, the Convention views disability as a product of the relationship between individuals and the barriers they face to participate in society on an equal basis with other citizens (11). In this sense, progress on improving rights and social participation requires addressing thc barriers which hinder persons with disabilities in their day to day lives.

For persons with disabilities, 'social inclusion' has been said to involve two core dimensions – participating as valued individuals in the social, economic, political and cultural life of the community, and being involved in mutually appreciative and respectful interpersonal relationships (12). This understanding is close to Nancy Fraser's (13) notion of social justice which the author equates with 'parity of participation'. In Fraser's model, equal participation requires economic justice, linked to resource redistribution; cultural justice, linked to social recognition and respect for differences; and political justice, conceptualized as the opportunity to make one's voice heard in society. All these dimensions are relevant to persons with disabilities who often face exclusion due to economic deprivation, social devaluation and lack of political voice. Yet, as argued by Pinto (14) to adequately acknowledge and address the different needs of persons with disabilities, a fourth dimension is required - the reconfiguration of physical and social environments to render them more inclusive of all people, regardless the nature of their impairments.

Building on this literature, a working definition of social inclusion was developed for the purpose of this study, focusing on three interconnected dimensions: a) access to the social, economic, political and cultural life of the community on equal terms with other citizens; b) access to material resources, adequate support and reasonable accommodation, so as to render that participation possible; and c) engagement in meaningful, rewarding and respectful interpersonal relationships.

OUR STUDY

This study relied on a mixed-methods approach, combining qualitative and quantitative procedures in a 'mutually enlightening' manner (15), through a triangulation of data sources (i.e., 285 questionnaires and 48 semi-structured interviews) and analytic procedures (i.e., descriptive and inferential statistics and content analysis), thereby minimizing the potential limitations of each method (16).

Sampling followed non-probabilistic procedures and developed in two stages. The first stage applied the Politz method (itinerary method). In the second stage, sampling was based on a quota procedure. Data from the

1998 and 2008 Population Census, published by the National Bureau of Statistics (ONS), concerning the distribution of types of impairments, age group and gender in the disabled population were used to define the quotas. The identification of the respondents followed a snowball procedure that started with the identification of participants through local disabled persons' organizations, as well as education and health services. Each participant was then invited to indicate other potential interviewees, which allowed the research team to reach people outside the services network.

Data collection proceeded also in two stages. First a questionnaire, adapted from an instrument created by Trani and colleagues, was applied, aimed to obtain a detailed account of the living conditions of persons with disabilities, aged 15-45 years-old, in the region of Algiers. The questionnaires assessed the socio-demographic and socio-economic profile of persons with disabilities living in the region and provided an initial analysis of the patterns concerning barriers to social inclusion and social participation. Data thus collected was analysed with SPSS, through procedures of descriptive and inferential statistics Chi square Independence Test for p=0,005).

Then, semi-structured interviews were conducted using an adapted version of the DRPI interview guide, a flexible tool to assess situations of discrimination and their human rights implications. The guide allowed interviewees to identify themselves the domains in which they had experienced greater barriers to social inclusion. Once a particular event, taking place over the course of the past five years, was identified a number of additional probing questions were asked, in order to explore in detail the situation and understand its human rights implications. Interviews were analysed using the NVivo-10 software. Content analysis identified the domains where the situation was experienced - Intimacy and Family Life; Education; Health and Rehabilitation; Work; Justice; Income Security and Support Services; Social Participation; and/or Information and Communication – as well as its implications for the fulfillment or denial of five human rights principles: Dignity; Autonomy; Inclusion, participation and accessibility; Equality and non-discrimination; and Respect for difference.

The data collection instruments were designed to be responded directly by the person with a disability and in private. Whenever the nature of the impairment did not allow the person with disability to respond to the questionnaire individually, the assistance of a third party, designated by the participant himself/herself, was sought. Most questionnaires were responded directly by persons with disabilities themselves (n=238), a minority with the assistance of a third party (n=12) or solely by a third party (n=35), mostly a family member or support staff. The qualitative part of the study (the 48 in-depth interviews) were conducted with persons with disabilities selected among the questionnaire respondents. All interviews were granted directly by the person with disability individually, without the presence of assistants.

FINDINGS

The 285 persons interviewed for this study included persons with physical (n=91), intellectual (n=78), visual (n=56), hearing (n=21) and multiple disabilities (n=39). Despite our efforts to ensure a balanced sampling, the sample suffered a gender and age bias. It was not possible, in the period available for data collection, to identify the established number of women willing to participate in the study, both due to lower levels of women's involvement in the organizations contacted and/or resistance expressed both by the women with disabilities themselves and by their family members (e.g., parents, husbands) to participate in the study, especially in light of the sensitive nature of the information that would be collected. Distribution by age group suffered a similar bias, with a higher ratio of younger participants, easier to identify through local organizations and services, suggesting different levels of social participation according to age group.

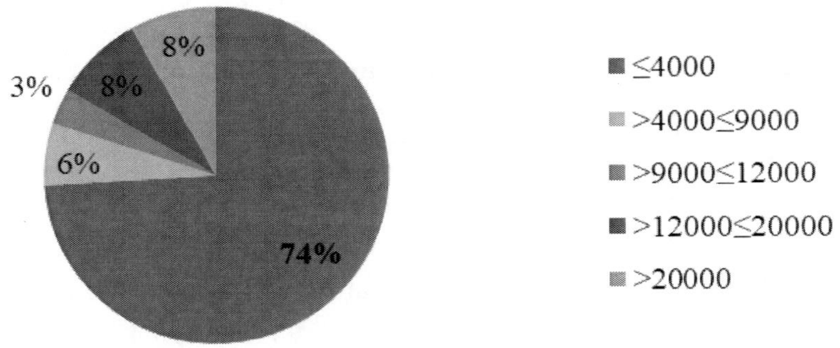

Figure 1. Distribution of the respondents by monthly income level (%).

Most respondents faced severe economic deprivation (see Figure 1). In fact, 74% of the respondents had a monthly individual income equal or below 4,000 Algerian dinars per month, the current value of the solidarity pension provided to persons with a complete incapacity to work and without any other revenue, bordering the level of absolute poverty as defined by the World Bank (1,25$ per day, corresponding to approximately 4,000 Algerian dinars per month, as per current exchange rate), whereas according to the National Bureau of Statistics, the average monthly income amounted to 36,100 Algerian dinars per month in 2013 (17).

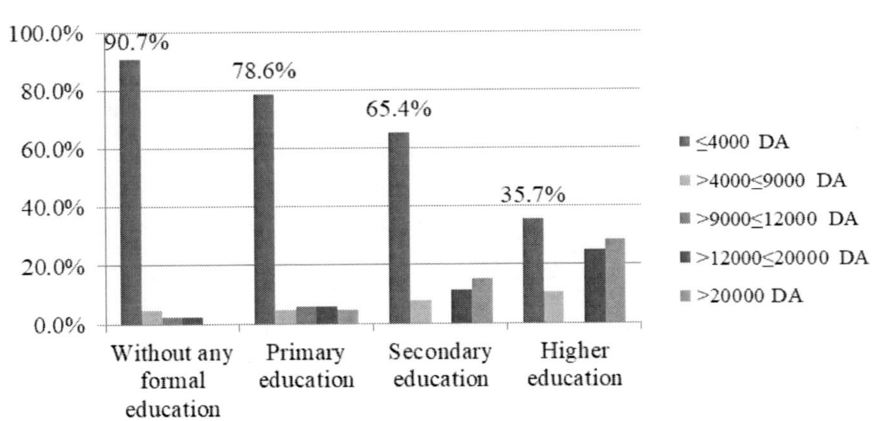

Figure 2. Relation between level of education and income level (%).

Moreover, an overview of the results of the questionnaire reveals that 21% of the participants did not have any formal education, the majority of the respondents (55%) only completed primary education, 12% secondary education and just 12% achieved higher education. As seen in figure 2, if education did not ensure, in itself, access to an adequate income, its absence seems to further compound the risk of economic exclusion: indeed 90.7% of those without any formal education are in the lowest level of income, contrasting with 35.7% among the higher educated group.

General trends concerning access and satisfaction with services

The questionnaire included a number of questions regarding access to and satisfaction with services. Figure 3 shows that public services are those where the greatest barriers were experienced (problems of access reported by 49% of the interviewees), closely followed by healthcare services (46%) and social services (37%).

The Chi Square Independence Test for a p value =0,005 did not reveal any significant gender or age group differences in barriers to access experienced. Nevertheless, significant differences were found concerning access to healthcare, public and employment services, in relation to type of disability (see Figure 4): lack of accessibility to healthcare services was mentioned mostly by people with physical (60%) or multiple impairments (62%), lack of access to social services by people with hearing or physical impairments (57% in each group) and lack of access to public services by people with physical (65%) or multiple impairments (64%).

The questionnaire also examined the level of general satisfaction or dissatisfaction with services. Figure 5 shows the services where the greatest levels of dissatisfaction were experienced.

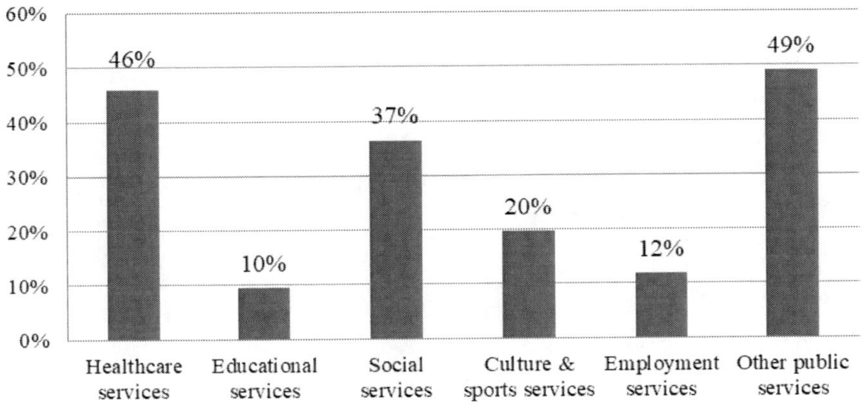

Figure 3. Respondents who reported lack of access to services by type of service (%).

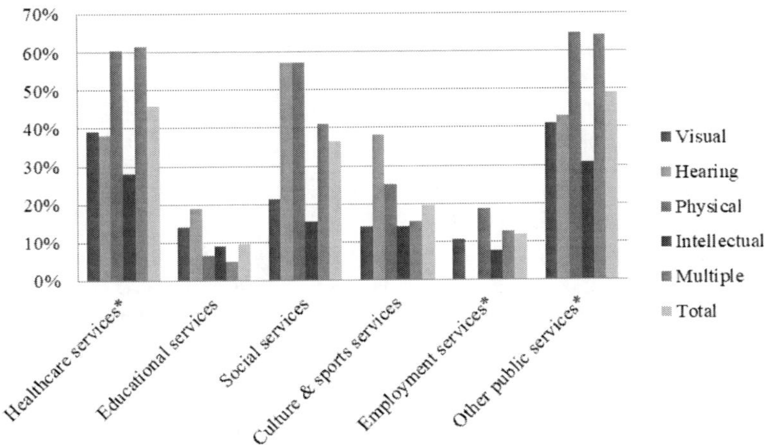

Figure 4. Percentage of respondents who reported lack of access to services by type of service and type of impairment (significant differences in a $\chi 2$ independence test for a p value $\leq 0{,}005$ marked with an *).

The Chi Square Independence Test for a p value =0,005 did not reveal any significant differences in levels of dissatisfaction with services on the basis of gender, but showed significant differences on the grounds of age and type of disability. Age proved to have a significant effect on the level of dissatisfaction with services for all services considered, with the greatest levels of dissatisfaction being expressed by people in the higher age groups (25-34 and 35-45) (see Figure 6).

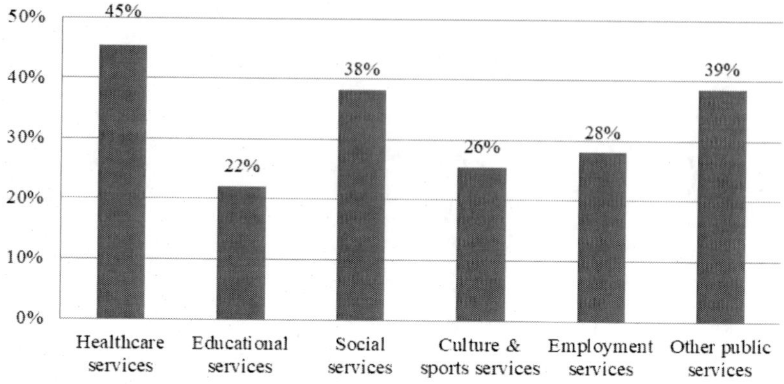

Figure 5. Percentage of respondents who reported dissatisfaction with services by type of service.

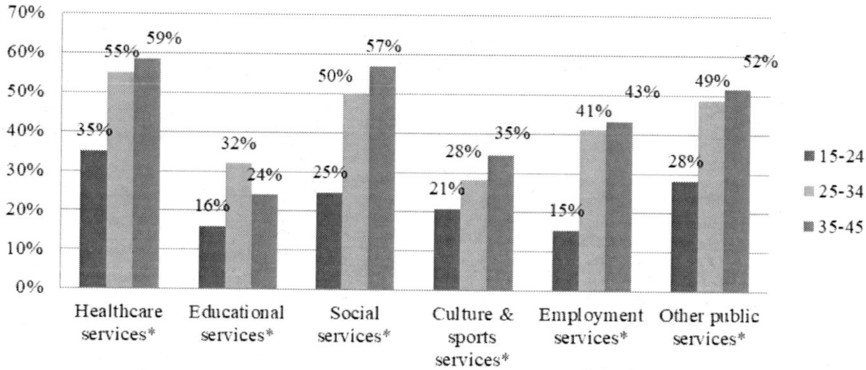

Figure 6. Percentage of respondents who reported dissatisfaction with services by type of service and age group (significant differences in a $\chi2$ independence test for a p value $\leq$0,005 marked with an *).

As for the type of impairment, significant differences were found concerning dissatisfaction with healthcare, social and culture and sports services, with the highest levels of dissatisfaction being expressed by people with hearing impairments (90% for healthcare services, 67% for social services and 57% for culture and sports services). The lowest levels of dissatisfaction were in every instance found among people with intellectual impairments (see Figure 7).

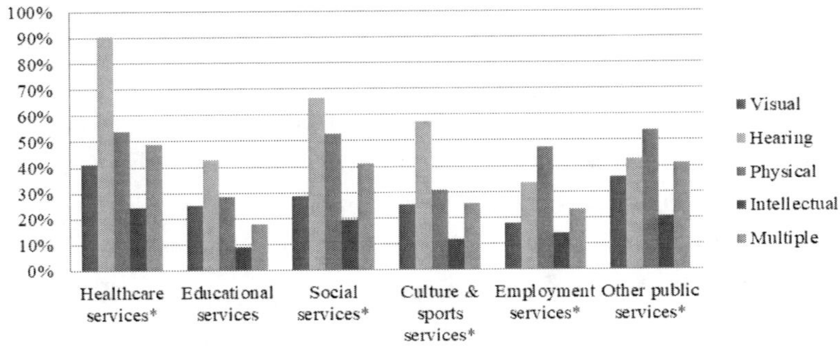

Figure 7. Percentage of respondents who reported dissatisfaction with services by type of service and type of disability (significant differences in a $\chi2$ independence test for a p value $\leq 0,005$ marked with an *).

Barriers to Social Inclusion

The in-depth interviews allowed the identification of life domains in which obstacles to social inclusion are most severely experienced. They were Social Participation (mentioned by 65% of the respondents), Intimacy and Family Life (mentioned by 35% of the respondents), Economic Security and Support Services and Work (both addressed by 25% of the respondents). For each of these domains, a description of the most important barriers to social inclusion will be presented in terms of their implications for the fulfillment of five cross-cutting human rights principles - Dignity, Autonomy, Participation, inclusion, and accessibility, Non-discrimination and equality, and Respect for difference. Dignity refers to the sentiment of being respected and valued in one's interaction with others; Autonomy indicates the ability to make decisions concerning one's life and obtaining the necessary support in order to do so; Participation, inclusion and accessibility encompasses being recognized as a full member in society, including through a barrier-free environment that enables full participation; Equality and Non-Discrimination means to have one's rights ensured in equal terms with other citizens, without distinction, exclusion or restriction on the grounds of disability; Respect for Difference implies being respected and having disability-related needs properly addressed.

Domain 1: Social participation

The domain of social participation encompassed all experiences of participation and interaction in community life, including access to cultural, sports, leisure and political activities.

Most barriers and denial of human rights in the domain of social participation included the absence of a positive attention to difference, as evidenced in the lack of accessibility of sidewalks, streets, public buildings, leisure facilities, and public transportation, or the lack of respect for priority in public transportation and other social situations. This lack of respect for difference also included direct negative attitudes towards persons with disabilities, such as staring, labeling, jockeying or insulting, as one of the interviewees confided:

> "A group of people I don't feel comfortable with tells me 'he's not a human being', 'he's an orphan', 'autistic'." (AF.AL.AL.A.09)

In some cases, lack of respect for difference prevented people from fully participating in social life, leading to situations of exclusion, as illustrated in the following example:

> "In the subway we find 60 steps, it's not made for someone with disability. Even if we find a passage for persons with disabilities, in order to get there, there are 20 steps! How am I supposed to go down?!" (AF.AL.AL.A.12)

These barriers to social participation also entail important consequences in regards to a sense of human dignity that is so often taken away from the person with disability:

> "Something that hurts me is the way people see me, as someone disabled… I feel a twinge of sadness, it hurts me. Their stare hurts me to the highest level… Yes, it's their look that breaks me!" (AF.AL.AL.A.23)

Domain 2: Intimacy and family life

This domain included all issues related to family and intimate life. Data from the interviews revealed important sociocultural barriers to inclusion of persons with disabilities in family life, particularly negative attitudes expressed by families of origin or families of prospective spouses that created important obstacles to the possibility of marriage and child-bearing. The human rights principles most affected by these situations were respect for difference and dignity:

> "Whenever I did something that did not please them, they [grandmother and father] would criticize and scold me. They would call me 'disabled' – my father described me that way and my grandmother as a trisomic child'. (AF.AL.AL.A.21 – Disrespect for Difference)

Intimacy and family life was also the domain that presented the paradoxical situation of being the domain where most situations of both inclusion and exclusion were reported. In other words, the way families welcomed or rejected disability-related differences played a vital role in the human rights experiences of persons with disabilities. Inclusion, for instance, was identified in reports of several activities done as a family and the efforts made by family-members to make the person with disability feel a part of the family group, as in the following example:

> [Interviewer: Your friends have left you?]
>
> "Yes, but my brother stays with me - we always go out together, we go for a walk together, we spend the evening at home together…There's a big difference between family and friends!" (AF.AL.AL.A.12)

Domain 3: Income security and support

This domain included all experiences related to economic security and support services. The key barriers reported in the interviews were attitudinal factors and bureaucratic obstacles that prevented effective access to social services and assistance. The most frequent human right implication was exclusion from access to social supports:

> "At first, I had access to a yellow card of 100% [official recognition of a total degree of incapacity], afterwards, they gave me 80%. I presented appeal 2 or 3 times… last time I protested they told me to be patient, that they would solve my situation after the elections… When my file passed by the [medical] commission they said 'you don't have the right to complaint'" (AF.AL.AL. C.01 - Exclusion)

Another frequently reported barrier concerns being disrespected when accessing services. Talking about the attitudes of public servants in a social services department one interviewee commented:

> "What do they do? Well, most of them don't welcome you or don't truly see you as someone who actually has a right. They make fun of you and play you along…" (AF.AL.AL.C.01 – Disrespect for Difference).

This disrespectful attitudes often had implications for the sense of personal dignity of those who had to endure them, as illustrated by the following example:

> "It hurts…it hurts my feelings… How could it not hurt you?! It hurts because if someone has their health and is capable, he doesn't need to deal with this person. In my case, it's because of my health I am in this situation… Some people will always remain inferior in the regard of others." (AF.AL.AL. C.01)

A further important implication concerned the lack of autonomy in the context of social services, reinforced by the negative attitudes of some professionals:

> "They don't consider me as a human being capable of sorting my papers or being responsible for myself and think I should let my father take me as his responsibility!" (AF.AL.AL.A.09 – Lack of Autonomy)

As this example suggests, denying the autonomy is just another way of devaluing the person and his/her humanity.

Domain 4: Work

The domain of work includes all experiences related to access to employment and the labour market. Most situations reported in the interviews referred to situations of discrimination or exclusion from employment opportunities, with important consequences to the sense of dignity of the interviewees, as in the following quotes:

> "He gave each person a different salary. (…) He paid the three others [persons with disabilities] and me always less." (AF.AL.AL.A.10 – Discrimination and Inequality)
>
> "At the factory they told me 'You cannot work, you have a disability'. (…) I asked for a trial period and they refused." (AF.AL.AL.A.01 - Exclusion)
>
> "I want to work, but I can't, people refuse me.... I feel useless... I ask myself 'Why was I born, why am I born useless?!'"(AF.AL.AL.A.23 – Violation of Dignity)

Given the importance of work to access an adequate income, as well as for social inclusion and human wellbeing, facing exclusion and discrimination in the labor market is a strong indicator of the marginal place that persons with disability still occupy in the Algerian society.

DISCUSSION

This chapter presented the results of a study that aimed to assess the barriers that hinder the social inclusion of persons with disabilities in Algiers. The concept of social inclusion adopted in this paper included three dimensions, namely: 1) Access to social, economic, political and cultural life on equal terms with other citizens; 2) Access to material resources, reasonable accommodation and other necessary support in order to facilitate this participation; 3) Involvement in interpersonal interactions that are significant and respectful of individual dignity. Results show that despite recent advances in the Algerian legal and policy framework, none of these conditions is yet fully satisfied for persons with disabilities in Algiers.

Specifically, results suggest two major types of obstacles to social inclusion. On one hand, there are a number of persisting macro and meso-level structural factors, such as inadequate implementation of existing legislation (for instance regarding accessibility and non-discrimination), lack of effective mechanisms of monitoring and enforcement of legal provisions (e.g., of the quota law for employment of persons with disabilities), and lack of access to independent and accessible complaint mechanisms. On the other hand, important micro-level sociocultural barriers (e.g., negative attitudes towards persons with disabilities, such as staring, mockery, lack of respect for priority, among others) render access to education, healthcare, employment, family life and all areas of social inclusion particularly difficult. Often, persons are subject to discrimination in various domains of everyday life, exacerbating feelings of exclusion. For instance, several interviewees reported having faced significant barriers during their educational path, which led them to early school drop-out and increased difficulties of inclusion in the labor market. These barriers help explain some of the indicators of social exclusion found among the target-group, particularly the low educational attainment levels (21% with no formal educational attainment level and 55% with just primary education), high economic vulnerability (74% with a monthly income bordering an absolute poverty level), high rates of exclusion from the labor market (33% either inactive or unemployed) and intimate relationships (90% single).

Taken together, these findings show that changes at the legal and policy level, while important, are only shifting sands, and remain insufficient to bring about deeper social change. Further research is needed to continue shed light on the sociocultural barriers, mechanisms and processes that prevent the successful implementation of current legislative and political commitments in order to address these barriers and improve the prospects of social inclusion of persons with disabilities, in Algeria and elsewhere.

ACKNOWLEDGMENTS

The authors would like to thank: Handicap International and the US-Middle East Partnership Initiative (MEPI), who funded this research in the scope of the project LEAD (2013-2014) and the Algerian Federation of Persons with Disabilities, key partners throughout the project, as well as Jean-François Trani and colleagues, who kindly shared data collection tools applied in the scope of the project LEAD Morocco and Tunisia.

REFERENCES

[1] Plateforme des Organisations Algériennes pour la mise en œuvre de la Convention relative aux Droits des Personnes Handicapées. Communication 2011. URL: http://lib.ohchr.org/HRBodies/UPR/Documents/session13/DZ/JS1_UPR_DZA_S13_2012_JointSubmission1_F.pdf.

[2] Pinto PC, Pinto TJ, Cunha A. L'inclusion sociale des personnes en situation de handicap dans la wilaya d'Alger. Alger: Handicap International – Programme Maghreb/Fédération Algérienne des Personnes Handicapées, 2014.

[3] Oyaro LO. Africa at Crossroads: The United Nations Convention on the Rights of Persons with Disabilities. Am Univ Int Law Rev2015;30(2):347-77.

[4] Bakhshi P, Gall F, Lopez D, Tani JF. Le handicap dans les politiques publiques tunisiennes face au creusement des inégalités et à l'appauvrissement des familles avec des ayants droit en situation de handicap. Tunis: Handicap International, 2014.

[5] Union of Physically Disabled Against Segregation (UPIAS). Fundamental principles of disability 1976. URL: http://disability-studies.leeds.ac.uk/files/library/UPIAS-fundamental-principles.pdf.

[6] Finkelstein V. Attitudes and disabled people: Issues for discussion 1980. New York: World Rehabilitation Fund, 1980. URL: http://disability-studies.leeds.ac.uk/files/library/finkelstein-attitudes.pdf.

[7] Oliver M. Social work with disabled people. Basingtoke: Macmillan, 1983.

[8] Jaeger P, Bowman C. Understanding disability: Inclusion, access, diversity and civil rights. Westport, CT: Praeger, 2005.

[9] Barnes C, Mercer G. Independent futures: Creating user led disability services in a disabling society. Bristol: Policy Press, 2006.

[10] Albrecht G, Ravaud JF, Stiker HJ. L'Émergence des disability studies: état des lieux et perspectives. Sci Soc Santé 2001;19(4):43-73.

[11] Mégret F. The Disabilities Convention: Human rights of persons with disabilities or disability rights? Human Rights Quart 2008;30:494-516.

[12] Roeher Institute Towards a common approach to thinking about and measuring social inclusion. Toronto, ON: Roeher Institute, 2003.

[13] Fraser N. Reframing justice in a globalizing world. New Left Rev 2005;36:69-88.

[14] Pinto P. Dilemas da Diversidade: Interrogar a deficiência, o género e o papel das políticas públicas em Portugal. Lisboa: Fundação Calouste Gulbenkian e Fundação para a Ciência e Tecnologia, 2012.

[15] Bryman A. Social research methods. Oxford: OUP, 2012.

[16] Maxwell J. Qualitative research design: An interactive approach. Thousand Oaks, CA: Sage, 1996.

[17] Office National des Statistiques. Résultats de l'enquête annuelle sur les salaires auprès des entreprises – Rapport n° 675. Alger: Office National des Statistiques - Direction technique chargée des statistiques sociales et des revenus, 2013.

In: Disability: International Aspects
Editors: Ariel Tenenbaum et al.
ISBN: 978-1-53617-886-9

Chapter 7

IMPLEMENTATION OF A NATIONAL POLICY FOR PERSONS WITH DISABILITIES IN CHANDIGARH, INDIA

Aditi Gupta[1,*], BDS, MPH, Amarjeet Singh[1], MBBS, MD and Ravneet Kaur[2], MBBS, MD

[1]School of Public Health, Post Graduate Institute of Medical Education and Research, Chandigarh, India

[2]Department of Community Medicine, All India Institute of Medical Sciences, New Delhi, India

ABSTRACT

The disability rights are being recognized around the world with legislations focusing on development of inclusive societies. Our study explores the relevance of a national policy for persons with disabilities in the city of Chandigarh, which is the best planned city in the northern part of India. To understand the extent of the implementation of policy, in-

---

* Corresponding Author: Aditi Gupta, Senior Research Officer, School of Public Health, Post Graduate Institute of Medical Education and Research, Sector 12, Chandigarh-160012, India. E-mail: dr.aditigupta86@yahoo.com.

depth interviews were conducted with officials of thirty government and private departments A checklist to get quantitative scores on disable friendliness of public places was also completed. Information available through secondary sources like official websites, government reports was also used to get the information. Policy implementation score was 60% which is on the lower limit of good score. This score can be considered low for a planned city like Chandigarh. We also found that some concerned officials were unaware of some of the provisions given to PWDs but were willing to know and implement it. Understanding the implementers' point of views is important for further planning strategies when world is aiming towards achievement of sustainable development goals (SDGs) that call for promotion of peaceful and inclusive societies.

INTRODUCTION

Disability is a condition which restricts a person's mental, sensory, or mobility functions to undertake or perform a task in the same way as a person who does not have a disability (1). The World Health Organization describes it as an umbrella term, which not only includes impairment but also activity limitation and participation restriction (2). It is estimated that 10% of the world's population had some kind of disability, and around 80% reside in rural areas (3). Only 2-3% persons with disabilities (PWD) could benefit from rehabilitation services in developing countries (3).

The census of 2001 showed that there were approximately 2.19 core persons with disabilities in India who constitute 2.13 percent of the total population (4). Out of this, only 49% were literate and only 34% were employed (4). The social model of disability explains that disability is imposed by society by excluding their participation and limiting their opportunities (5). The noble laureate Amartya Sen has used the term "conversion handicap," whereby people with disabilities derive a lower level of welfare from a given level of income than the rest of population; due to additional costs incurred in converting income into wellbeing. However, the rights of PWDs are now being recognized around the world and many disability related legislations are coming into being at international, national and state levels (6).

In India, there are many legislations related to disabilities including the Mental Health Act 1987 (7), The Rehabilitation Council Act of India (RCI, 1992) (8), The Persons with Disabilities (Equal Opportunities, Full Participation and Protection of Rights) Act 1995 (9), The National Trust (For welfare of persons with Autism, Cerebral Palsy, Mental Retardation and Multiple Disabilities) Act, 1999 (10). The National Policy for Persons with Disabilities (NPPWD) was announced in year 2006 which seeks to create an environment that provides basic principles of equality, freedom, justice and dignity for all individuals including the persons with disabilities as mentioned in the constitution of India (11).

However, effective implementation of any policy determines its success and failure rates (12). Policy implementation is a complex process which requires sophisticated interaction and coordination both within and between different sectors (13). Despite decades of existence of such legislations, there is a lack of evidential support in literature to see the extent of implementation of these policies (14-16). Thus, the present study was undertaken to evaluate the implementation of the National Policy for Persons with Disabilities (NPPWD) as well as to access opinion of implementers' towards policy provisions in Chandigarh city.

OUR STUDY

This cross sectional study was conducted in 2013-14 in the Union Territory of Chandigarh situated in northern part of which has 1.05 million population in an area of 114 km^2 (17). The primary unit of city's design is a sector, which is 800 x 1,200 meters in area (17). Chandigarh has 56 sectors, 18 villages (13 in rural belt and 5 under Municipal Cooperation) and 41 slums. To understand the extent of implementation, the policy was divided into various domains and under each domain departments responsible for providing key services was recognized. More than 30 public and private departments/offices/organizations were visited and the officials were contacted to get the required information. Some data and information was also collected from the official websites of Chandigarh administration and internet. The domain names along with list of government offices visited under them are mentioned in Table 1.

Table 1. Summary table for the policy domains and their scores

Domain No.	Name	Department Visited	Score Obtained (Max.)	Percentage
1)	Responsibility for Implementation of the policy	Department of Social Welfare,	2/(6)	33.33%
2)	Prevention, early diagnosis and intervention	Department of Social Welfare, Department of Education, Community health centers, Rehabilitation centers and NGOs	8/(10)	80%
3)	Physical Rehabilitation	Department of Social Welfare Rehabilitation centers and NGOs	8/(10)	80%
4)	Human Resource Development	Department of Social Welfare	5/(8)	62.5%
5)	Education	Department of Education, Department of Social Welfare Government and private schools, Resource centre for PWDs, Rehabilitation centers, National Institute for Teacher Training and Research	15/(22)	68.18%
6)	Economic Rehabilitation	Department of Social Welfare, National Handicapped Finance and Development Corporation, Government and Private Banks	8/(11)	72.72%
7)	Barrier Free environment	Department of Social Welfare	5.5/(11)	50%
8)	Social Protection	Department of Social Welfare	10 /(17)	58.82%
9)	Research	Department of Science and Technology, Central Scientific Instrumentation Organization, National Institute for Teacher Training and Research	3.5/(10)	35%
10)	Sports, Recreation and Cultural activities	Department of Sports, Department of Tourism, Markets, Malls, Public Parks, Tourist places,	1 /(5)	20%
	Final Score		66 /(110)	60%

Data collection and analysis

The data collection was done during months of May-June, 2014 by the authors. Prior permissions and appointments were taken from governmental and nongovernmental organizations. An assessment tool and scoring system was developed based on the provisions mentioned under different domains of the policy. The tool was pretested and necessary changes were made in the tool to collect data.

For scoring each question in the assessment tool carried the equal score of one. Scoring system was fully dependent on the provisions of policy, if any provision of NPPWD was found available in Chandigarh, then it was scored one otherwise it was counted as zero. For calculating the finest score for each item, unitary method was used. A grading system was developed to interpret the final score. There were total ten domains carrying 110 items each carrying a score of two, making a total score of 110 (see appendix). A grading scheme was developed dividing the scores in five grades, viz., excellent (80-100%), good (60-79.9%), average (40-59.9%), poor (20-39.9%) and very poor (0-19.9%). Departments responsible for provisions under different domains were visited to understand the implementation level. The authorities accountable were interviewed. Some data was also collected from the official website of Chandigarh Administration and were counter checked in the interviews. The study employed a range of qualitative methods like in-depth interviews, observations, secondary literature search etc. Along with obtaining the information from the officials, we also explored the ground reality by visiting the sites like markets, stadiums, recreational centers, research institutes, training centers etc. A checklist to get quantitative scores on disable friendliness of public places was also completed.

Ethical approval and consent

The ethical approval was obtained from the Institute Ethical Committee of Post Graduate Institute of Medical Education and Research. Permission for conducting the study was obtained from the Department of Social Welfare, Chandigarh administration. All the interviews were conducted after obtaining written permissions from the officials of the concerned department of Chandigarh administration.

FINDINGS

For the first objective, ten domains were developed under the policy provisions. These were Identification of policy stakeholders; prevention, early diagnosis and intervention; rehabilitation programme, human resource development, education, economic rehabilitation, barrier-free environment, social protection, research and sports, recreation and cultural activities.

A total thirty departments were visited to get the pertinent information. The cumulative score for Chandigarh in implementation of policy 66 out of 110 points i.e., 60%. Prevention, identification and diagnosis of disability (80%), physical rehabilitation (80%) and economic rehabilitation (72.72%) domains were the top three scoring domains. The domains scoring less than 60% are Sports and Recreation (20%), Identification of stakeholders (33.33%), Research (35%), Barrier free Environment (50%) and Social security (58.82%). Table 1 illustrates the combined scores obtained under various provisions. The questionnaire and detailed scoring under each domain is described in 'appendix1'.

The interviews conducted with various government and non government officials were translated and transcribed and were kept anonymous. The interviews highlighted the opinion and sensitization levels of officials towards achieving the barrier free and inclusive society for PWDs. In his words, the principal of a Blind School beautifully described the gist of our whole study in one line:

> "It is not the disability which is important in a disabled person……But it is the person who is important in a person with disability."

Early identification and prevention of disability

Regarding prevention of disability, the official website of National Health Mission, Chandigarh administration showed that various health programmes have performed well in the year 2012-2013. The National Program for Control of Blindness had achieved well above their set yearly targets (2012-2013) of surgeries, eye donations etc. (18). The prevalence rate of leprosy in Chandigarh reached less than 1 case in 1,000 in 2009, four years before the study was conducted (19). Similarly, no case of polio has been recorded after 2010.

For early identification and prevention of disability, training modules are present for teachers, anganwadi workers (AWW), auxillary nurse midwives (ANMs), medical and paramedical graduates. We interviewed five AWWs and ANMs each; it showed that their training for early identification of disabilities were not satisfactory. They were able to recognize the gross disabilities of limbs, eyes and mental abilities but lacked the knowledge for prevention of disabilities. There was only one AWW who had an idea about the rehabilitation facilities for PWDs, other than medical rehabilitation. This showed that our health workers are dedicated to community health but lack appropriate knowledge about rehabilitation. Our policy does not focus on the health promotion as a preventive measure. However, most of the disabilities are preventable.

Physical rehabilitation

The services for physical rehabilitation include medical rehabilitation & counseling along with vocational trainings. The city has a State Resource Center cum District Disability Rehabilitation Center and numerous other government and non government rehabilitation centers. There are many NGOs working for various disabilities in the city. The government has been working in collaboration with these NGOs to carry out various activities like providing aids and appliances at subsidized rates.

Assistive enabled devices (AEDs) are available at various tertiary care hospitals and rehabilitation centers in the city. People from urban area had easy access to aids and appliances while people living in slums faced maximum problem in free access to aids and appliances due to their ignorance about their rights towards facilities and provision under the policy.

Though the Chandigarh administration has been executing most of the points mentioned in the national policy, our visit to various rehabilitation centers showed that there was a shortage of human resources. For example, one renowned rehabilitation center whose daily OPD was in hundreds had only one physiotherapist. The manager of the center quoted, "we have 20,000 children registered in our rehabilitation center. Everyday hundreds of children come here but we have only one physiotherapist." There was a lack of regular assessment from the administration regarding requirement of human resources in rehabilitation centers.

A teacher in one of the rehabilitation center pointed out at the lack of age targeted interventions for disability," We do not have separate rehab centers for older people. Their demands are different from that of kids. Also, Counseling is still not considered an integral part of medical rehabilitation which is important to boost their confidence and self esteem.

Economic rehabilitation

The government has a reservation of three percent in all categories of jobs in the government sector and a strategy of giving incentives to private sector employers for promoting employment of people with disabilities. The data from the website of Statistics Department Chandigarh shows that NHFDC gave loans to 43 beneficiaries to a tune of 4.89 lakhs during 2006-2007 in Chandigarh (20). Equal division of the amount among beneficiaries showed that approximately 11 thousand rupees were given as loan to each recipient. Whether the amount provided was enough could not be assessed as the effect these strategies on actual financial condition of PWDs has never been evaluated.

Educational rehabilitation

The policy describes education as the most effective medium of social and economic empowerment. The study results showed excellent implementation of the educational provisions of the policy. It appeared that the government schools were doing well for integrating Children with special needs (CWSN) into the mainstream education while score of the private schools were poor. There were five resource centers in the city while the total number of government schools in Chandigarh was 107 (official data 2012-2013) from Department of Education, Chandigarh (21) Thus, there is one resource center for around 21 schools while the guidelines by RCI say that the ratio of resource center to schools should be 1:10 (22).

Along with resource centers, there was a shortage of resource teachers as well. There were only 14 resource teachers who are in-charge of training teachers about disability and providing home based education to bed ridden children around the city. The adverse ratio can affect the quality of services delivered. During interview, a resource teacher quoted," we have very less number of resource teachers. The ratio of a resource teacher specialized in mental disabilities to mentally challenged children is around 1:128. The same teacher cannot make more than 7-8 visits to a school in a year." The guidelines by Rehabilitation Council of India (RCI) demands availability of specialized teachers for each disability in every school. We observed that there was only one teacher in every government school who was taking care of each type of disability while there was no teacher trained in disability in the private school.

Our interview with the principal of a government school highlighted that two children with physical disability were dropped out of school due to their aggressive nature. On asking reason, she quoted" when a child is aggressive, he can injure other kids. We called their parents and told them if the child would not behave properly, they might be expelled." The children were not counseled for their behaviour. Although the fact cannot be generalized on the basis of one interview but the case demonstrated that the sensitization training of teachers and principals was found wanting.

Barrier free environment

The sign boards pertaining to PWD were missing at all the public places visited. The policy directs the governments to put up sign boards at all the public places for PWDs. Many places had ramps but in the absence of appropriate sign boards, they were being easily missed by the wheelchair users. The ramp at the entrance of Chandigarh Railway Station and Sector 17 Interstate Bus Tribunal (ISBT) were appropriate for wheelchair users. However, a wheel chair user could not board him to train. The low floor buses which were considered disabled friendly by the administration did not have extendable ramps from the bus floors. However, seats were reserved for PWDs in public transport.

The roads also need to be designed for safe and hassle free movement of disabled persons. Nowhere can one find curb cuts, guiding blocks. The cuts were present at the zebra crossings but they lack proper designs. Random selection of markets and public parking showed absence of separate parking areas for PWDs.

Most of the markets in Chandigarh are multi storied and have steps before the markets making them disabled unfriendly. Some markets have disabled friendly toilets. But these were either locked or were not in proper working conditions. Most of the ATMs in the city lacked the audio support required for blind persons except some private banks.

Welfare

The websites of Chandigarh Administration lack screen reading technologies and are not accessible to visually impaired. This implies that a blind person cannot avail the information online independently. All the public documents are also not available in Braille and tape recordings. This shrinks their pool for getting information.

A provision provides free transport facilities to physically and mentally challenged individuals within union territory of Chandigarh. A random interview with the bus conductor of Chandigarh Transport Unit on the local bus stand showed their ignorance about the provision," assi taan bas 12 saal to khat bacche di ya buzurg bande di aadhi ticket katde haan, aur kise di ni." (We only cut the half ticket for children less than 12 years old or senior citizens and no one else).

The IEC materials like booklets and charts etc are available mostly at the official websites, offices and the concerned departments. They are not accessible at the public places where they are more advantageous to the common people. The social security nets for disabled women are all the more important as a disabled woman is more vulnerable to sexual and physical abuse. The city lacked separate hostels for the disabled girls with every kind of disability.

For addressing the concern of lack of information sources, Chandigarh Administration has started a helpline for PWD, (Helpline number is 108) where they can call in case of emergency, abuse or for seeking concerned information.

Research

A lot of research work is undergoing on the topic of disability in the city but none of the research institute was working under the local administration. All the research is being financed through the central government. An official from Science and Technology Department said, "Our department had nothing to do with disability. It is the work area of CSIO, another institute in the city." On the contrary the policy says that it is the responsibility of the Ministry of Science and Technology to set up Rehabilitation Technology Center for undertaking research in testing and certifying trainings and new technologies. This showed that research in disability was a low priority area for the administration. The reason can be indifferent attitude, lack of instruction/awareness or lack of answerability to public.

Sports and tourism

These were among the least scoring domains in our study. Sport is only seen as a recreational activity and not as a career for PWDs in the city. On asking about the reason for the lack of initiatives from the sports department, the official expressed his helplessness by quoting, "we cannot do anything alone. The Department of Social Welfare should give us some guidelines, we will be happy doing work on disability. We help our disabled players who bring medals for us by giving them money. Separate coach is not available." A tourism officer quoted: "The idea of working for disability never came to our mind. This is a very novel idea. We will discuss it"

DISCUSSION

This study was the first initiative of its kind to evaluate the extent to which a national policy for persons with disabilities had been implemented in a city in India. Our study revealed despite being the best planned city of the country, the score for level of implementation was just 60% which falls on lower side of the good grade.

Chandigarh, the dream city of India's first Prime Minister, Sh. Jawahar Lal Nehru, was planned by the famous French architect Le Corbusier. It is known as one of the best experiments in urban planning and modern architecture in the twentieth century in India. It was the first planned city of Independent India. As per census 2011, the literacy rate of the city is 86.43% (23). It has also been ranked first in Human Development Index and Gender Development Index, Greenery and Plantation, Purity of Drinking Water, efficiency of Garbage Disposal, Cleanliness of public toilets, participation of Municipality, Cleanliness on roads and Dustbin in public places by far in the country by ORG-AC Nielson in their recent survey (24). City also has an extensive network of health facilities, educational institutes, research institutes, etc. therefore Chandigarh can be described as the first model city of the country (17). Hence, it is expected that the city should home the best facilities in every sphere of our lives. In context of our studies also it is expected that implementation of policy for PWDs would be excellent.

Our inquiries revealed that the city has not framed any policy or specific rules for the disabled persons. However, it has implemented various national acts and regulations related to disability and recently declared its citizen charter (25). The performance of the policy for PWD was evaluated from the providers' perspective, so the results should have been a lot better.

Our study highlighted the role of inter-sectoral coordination among different stakeholders for the successful execution of the policy. As described earlier the NPPWD involves effective working among various government and non-government departments (11). In our study we found that though different departments were playing their defined roles but there was a lack of communication between them. Also, there had been no inter-departmental meeting on the issue of disability in the city in the last one year i.e., during financial year of 2012-13.

It was also felt that some provisions in the NPPWD are vague. For instance, the provision 51(ix) in the Barrier Free Environment 'encourages banking system to meet the needs of PWDs'. The context of the point is not clear as what actual role a bank should be playing. Similarly, for provision 53(i) to 53(vi) in research, it is not mentioned as which department would be responsible for it (11). The policy has not mentioned anything about social issues like stigma and discrimination attached to disability in our society. The provision of inclusive education cannot prevent dropout of CWSN facing negative labeling like Kaani, langdi, pagli (derogatory words in Hindi for PWDs) in schools. Even 3% reservation in jobs cannot ensure that a blind would not be refused a job in the local shops. Our study found that social attitudes and norms were among the major barrier in the lives of differently able people. The stigma restricts their participation in daily life activities like education, employment, social gatherings. Participation restrictions further push them towards seclusion, depression and poverty thus making it a vicious circle. Unfriendly physical infrastructure along with limited social access further worsens the condition of a disabled. Responsibility of a government lies in providing the right infrastructure and environment for their free movement. Until they can move around freely, all the provisions cannot be utilized properly. The policies should be extensive and explanatory as huge amount of resources are spent in laying down any infrastructure and once laid it remain there for a long time. So resources need to be utilized keeping in mind its future benefits. The top-down approach of programme formation and implementation should be replaced with more horizontal approach where PWDs are key stakeholders in the entire process and not merely passive recipients. The verbatim responses from the officials showed the need to sensitize and take the issue which was on desk for more than 18 years. The reversal of leprosy rates in recent years in the city further exaggerates the need to reinforce the efforts done. The importance of the drive for disability rights have further increased in last ten years as the census of 2011 showed a 22.4% total decadal growth of disabled population with an addition of 4.9 million PWDs to the numbers present in 2001 census. The urban disabled population showed an increase from 1.93% to 2.17% from 2001 to 2011 with a 55% decadal growth (26). India ratified the UN Convention on Rights of Persons with Disabilities (UNCRPD) in 2009 (27). However, passage of new Disability bill, 2016 is a step towards disability rights and a realization towards empowering this large section of society as a potential Vote Bank. The new law is supposed to not only boost the PWD rights but also provide effective mechanism for ensuring an inclusive and just society for them. Thus, there is further need for extensive research in field of policy implementation for PWDs to have their holistic involvement in the society.

ACKNOWLEDGMENTS

Financial disclosure: No funding obtained from any source. Data availability: All relevant data are within the paper and its supporting information files. Competing interests: No competing interests exist.

REFERENCES

[1] Australian Institute of Health and Welfare. Australian Government, Reasonable adjustments (Disability Discrimination Act) policy and procedures. URL: http://www.aihw.gov.au/WorkArea/DownloadAsset.aspx?id=60129552880.

[2] World Health Organization. Towards a common language for functioning, disability and health ICF, 2002. URL: http://www.who.int/classifications/icf/training/icfbeginnersguide.pdf.

[3] World Health Organization. World Bank Group, World report on disability, 2011. URL: http://www.who.int/disabilities/world_report/2011/report.pdf.

[4] Chavan B, Rozatkar AR. Intellectual disability in India: Charity to right based. Indian J Psychiatry 2014;56(2):113.

[5] O'Keefe P. People with disabilities from India: from commitments to outcomes. Human Development Unit, South East Asia Region. Washington, DC: World Bank, 2007:157.

[6] United Nations, Convention on the Rights of Persons with Disabilities and Optional Protocol. URL: http://www.un.org/disabilities/documents/convention/convoptprot-e.pdf.

[7] Ministry of Health and Family Welfare, Department of Health and Family Welfare, The Mental Health Act, 1987. URL: http://www.mohfw.nic.in/index1.php?lang=1&level=3&sublinkid=5196&lid=3184.

[8] The Rehabilitation Council act of India, 1992. URL: http://svayam.com/pdf/the_rci_act-1992&amendement_act_2000.pdf.

[9] The Persons With Disabilities (Equal Opportunities, Protection Of Rights And Full Participation) Act, 1995. URL: http://www.disabilityaffairs.gov.in/upload/upload files/files/PWD_Act.pdf.

[10] Ministry of Social Justice & Empowerment, Government of India, The National Trust (For welfare of persons with Autism, Cerebral Palsy, Mental Retardation and Multiple Disabilities) Act, 1999. URL: http://thenationaltrust.gov.in/upload/upload files/files/National%20Trust%20Act%20-%20Englsih.pdf.

[11] Minister Of Social Justice and Empowerment, Government of India, National Policy for Persons with Disabilities, 2006. URL: https://www.ilo.org/dyn/natlex/docs/ELECTRONIC/93612/109496/.../IND93612.pdf.

[12] McConnell A. Policy success, policy failure and grey areas in-between. J Public Policy 2010;30(03):345-62.

[13] Cerna L. The nature of policy change and implementation: a review of different theoretical approaches. Paris: Organisation for Economic co-opertion and development (OECD), 2013.

[14] Orton L, Lloyd WF, Taylor RD, O'Flaherty M, Capewell S. The use of research evidence in public health decision making processes: systematic review. PloS One 2011;6:7.

[15] Liverani M, Hawkins B, Parkhurst JO. Political and institutional influences on the use of evidence in public health policy. A systematic review. PLoS One. 2013;8(10):e77404.

[16] Hallsworth M. Policy-making in the real world. Political Insight 2011;2(1):10-2.

[17] Chandigarh the City Beautiful, The official website of Chandigarh Administration. URL: http://chandigarh.gov.in/.

[18] National Programme for Control of Blindness. State wise targets and achievement for various eye diseases during 2012-13. URL: http://npcb.nic.in/writeread data/mainlinkfile/File292.pdf.

[19] Department of Public Relations, Chandigarh Administration. Press release. Leprosy's total cure rate touches 100 per cent mark. 2009. URL: http://admser.chd.nic.in/uploadfiles/press/pressnote/pr6026.pdf.

[20] Department of Social Welfare, Chandigarh Administration. Statistics. URL: http://www.socialwelfare-tab28-1.pdf.

[21] Department of Education, Chandigarh Administration. URL: http://www.chdeducation.gov.in/schoolslist.asp.

[22] Sreekumari A. Evaluating the outcomes of inclusive education: A case study from India. Paper presented in International Conference on Inclusive Education. URL: www.ied.edu.hk/csnsie/resources/proceedings2003/proc17.pdf

[23] Demographic Profile of the City. Chandigarh master plan, 2031. URL: http://chandigarh.gov.in/cmp2031/demography.pdf.

[24] Jamshedpur ranks 2nd in 'quality of life' survey next to Chandigarh. URL: http://www.dailypioneer.com/state-editions/ranchi/jamshedpur-ranks-2nd-in-quality-of-life-survey.html.

[25] Social Welfare Department. Chandigarh Administration. Citizen charter. URL: http://chandigarh.gov.in/pdf/citizen_charter_sw.pdf.

[26] Office of the Registrar General and Census Commissioner, India. Census of India 2011: Data on disability. URL: http://www.censusindia.gov.in/2011census/Disability_Data/Disability_2011_Data_Release_Dec_2013_PPT%20(27.12.13).ppt.

[27] PRS Legislative research. The rIght of persons with disabilities bill. URL: http://www.prsindia.org/billtrack/the-right-of-persons-with-disabilities-bill-2014-3122/.

APPENDIX. SUPPLEMENTARY INFORMATION

Status of implementation of National Policy for Persons with Disabilities

Each question carried equal marks. For availability/presence, a full score of 1 is given and for absence, the score was 0. For partial availability, a score of 0.5 was given.

MOV= Mode of Verification

Responsibility for implementation of the policy

Policy involves various stakeholders for setting up necessary mechanism for implementation of the policy.

Provision/ Q. No	Evaluation Parameter	Availability (yes/no)	Score Obtd.
56/1	Presence of a nodal department for coordinating matters for implementation of the policy.*	Yes	1
57/2	Presence of District level committees including all stakeholders for coordinating implementation.	No	0
59/3	Chief commissioner for disability present.	Yes	1
60/4	Have Panchayats added the disability related components in their projects? **	No	0
62./5	Is there a state policy for persons with disabilities	No	0
62./6	If a comprehensive review of the policy is done every five years.	No	0
	Total (6)	2/6 = 33.3%	

*Department of Social Welfare is the nodal department working for implementation of the policy.
MOV--Q1, 2, 3, 5, 6 (Department of social welfare).
--Q4(The Action Plan for 12th FYP (2012-2017) available on the website of Rural Development and Panchayat Department did not mention about disability.)

Prevention, early diagnosis and intervention

Most of the disabilities are preventable if steps can be taken at the initial stages of the life. Early diagnosis and treatment can limit the extent of the disability.

Provision/ Q.No.	Prevention, early diagnosis and intervention	Availability	Score obtained
43(i)./07	Health programmes for immunization of children and expectant mothers, public health and sanitation	Yes	1
43(ii)./08	Regular training of medical and para- medical personnel for early identification and intervention.	Yes	1
43(iii)/09	Training modules for medical, paramedical and AWW for prevention and early diagnosis & interventions.	Yes	1
43(iv)/10	Training programmes and modules for postgraduate, undergraduate and diploma in medical education for disability prevention	No	0
43(v)./11	Disability specific manuals to families of PWDs	No	0
43(vi)./12	Human resource development institutions present in city.*	Yes	1
43(viii)/13	Development of plan of action for limiting disabilities within existing healthcare systems.	Yes	1
43(ix)./14	Awareness programmes for adolescent girls, mothers and women in reproductive age.	Yes	1
43(ix)./15	Awareness programmes for prevention of disability at level of teacher's training course.	Yes	1
43(x)./16	Screening programme for children in anganwadi and schools.	Yes	1
	Total score(10)		8 (80%)

*PGIMER develops human resources in physiotherapy, audiology, speech therapy, psychology etc.
MOV-Q7,14,15,16-(Department of Health, NRHM Chandigarh)
-Q8,9-(Medical Officer, PHC and AWW)
- Q10 (Postgraduate student, Pediatrics and Graduate student, Physiotherapy)
- Q11,12-(Department of Social Welfare)

Programme of rehabilitation

It includes medical rehabilitation & counseling, availability of Assistive devices and development of rehabilitation professionals.

Provision/ Q.No	Evaluation parameter	Availability (yes/no)	Score
	Medical and Physical Rehabilitation		
12./17	Physical rehabilitation measures like drugs, counseling, therapies and surgeries available at the major healthcare and rehab centers in the city.	Yes	1
11./18	Measures for disseminating information about facilities at rehabilitation centers to rural areas.	No	0
44 (I)/19	State Centers for composite rehabilitation services like human resource development, research.	Yes	1

Provision/ Q.No	**Evaluation parameter**	**Availability (yes/no)**	**Score**
44(ii)/20	Establishment of community based rehabilitation programmes.	Yes	1
44(iii)/21	Mental health care homes/ Custodial care institutions	Yes	1
44(iv)/22	Residential rehabilitation centers for vocational and social skill training for persons with mental illness.	Yes	1
	Assistive devices and rehabilitation professionals		
17./23	Free availability of aids and appliances through government/NGOs	Yes	1
18./24	Financial support by banks to manufacturers of the assistive devices.	Yes	1
19./25	Regular assessment of human resource requirements in rehabilitation.	No	0
20. /26	Rehabilitation centers for all kinds of disabilities.	Yes	1
	Total		8/10(80%)

MOV- Q17 to 26 (Annual Report of the Department of Social Welfare).

Human resource development

Trained Human resource is required for carrying out the rehabilitation process effectively.

Provision/ Q.no	**Evaluation parameter**	**Availability**	**Score obtained**
45(i)/27	Training of AWW and ANM in healthcare and community development for disability.	Yes	1
45(ii)/28	Support for training and orientation of personnel of government and NGO providing services.	Yes	1
45(iii)/29	Training and sensitization of community decision makers like panchayats and family heads	No	0
45(iv)/30	Training and orientation of family members as care givers.	No	0
46/31	Human resource training for inclusive, home based, special and preschool education.	Yes	1
46(i)/32	Training modules for teachers for inclusive education	Yes	1
46(ii)/33	Diploma, degree and high level programmes in special education	Yes	1
46(iii)/34	Training of caregivers for home based education and for disabled adults.	No	0
	Total (8)	5/8 = 62.5%	

MOV--Q27,28 (Department of Health), financial support and trainings at GMCH, Sector 32.
--Q29, 30- (Interview with a Resource teacher.)
--Q31,32,33,34- (Department of Education)

Education of persons with disabilities

The Department of Education was visited to collect the information about the mainstreaming of the persons with disabilities with regard to education.

Provision/ Q.No.	Educational rehabilitation	Availability (yes/no)	Score obtained
48(i)/35	Barrier free schools and colleges (building, toilets, labs etc.)	No	0
iii)/36	Resource centers as per ratio specified by RCI.*	No	0
iv)/37	Teaching aids and learning tools(Braille, talking books etc.)	No	0
v)/38	National Open schools and distance learning programmes	Yes	1
vi)/39	AAC (sign language, alternative and augmentative communication) in educational institutes.	No	0
vii)/40	Free mobility and support services provided.**	Yes	1
viii)/41	Parent teacher counseling and grievance redressal system***	No	0
ix)/42	steps for promoting education among disabled girl students at elementary, secondary and higher secondary education.#	Yes	1
x)/43	Special schools available for Children with Special Needs	Yes	1
xi)/44	Home based Education system	Yes	1
xii)/45	Modification of course curriculum and Examination systems.	Yes	1
xiii)/46	Inclusive pattern of education being followed	Yes	1
xiv)/47	Use of computers and technology in education of CWSN	No	0
xv)/48	Identification of children with disabilities up to 6 years of age by regular surveys and their training for inclusive education.	Yes	1
xvi)/49	Education for mentally ill persons in psychosocial centers	Yes	1
xvii)/50	Sensitization of teachers and principal to disability issues	Yes	1
xix)/51 xx)/52	Adult leisure and learning centers 3% reservation given in higher educational institutes	No Yes	0 1
xxi)/53	In service disability training programmes for teachers	Yes	1
21./54	Free education up to age of 18 years as specified by IEDC.	Yes	1
23./55	100% financial assistance to students for books, uniform etc.	Yes	1
25./56	Scholarships to disabled students during school and after to pursue higher studies.	Yes	1
	Total (22)	15/22= 68.18%	

* There were 5 Resource centers for 107 schools; while the RCI guidelines mention it to be 1 for 10 schools.

** Traveling and escort allowance worth 3000 rupees is given to students with disabilities.

***no psychological counseling sessions at parent- teacher meetings at schools.

a stipend of 200 rupees is given to girl students with disabilities for attending school.

MOV—Q35-56- (Department of Education);

Q36*- calculated by self;

Q41, 47-- (Principal of a Government School.)

Economic rehabilitation of PWDs

Employment opportunities available to the PWDs in government establishments, self employment etc were assessed by interviewing the Director, Department of Social Welfare and NHFDC (National Handicapped Finance and Development Corporation) and by visiting two banks.

Policy Provision	Employment for Persons with disabilities	Availability (Yes/no)	Score obtained
28(i)/57	3% reservation to PWD in government jobs.	Yes	1
28 (i)/58	Reservation is given in group A, B, C and D.	Yes	1
28(ii)/59	Incentives, awards, tax exemptions to the employers employing PWDs?	Yes	1
28(iii)/60	Tax concessions and exemption from duties to PWD?	Yes	1
28(iii)/61	Subsidized loans to PWDs by NHFDC or banks.	Yes	1
28(iii)/62	Financial support by NHFDC to self help groups	Yes	1
50(i)/63	Dialogues with private sector for creating employment opportunities for PWDs.	No	0
50(ii)/64	Development of Home based Income Generation Programmes for PWDs.	Yes	1
50(iii)/65	Modification of designing of machinery, workstation and work environment for PWDs	No	0
50(iv)/66	Assistance in marketing of goods produced by PWDs	Yes	1
50(v)/67	Coverage of PWDs in various poverty alleviation programs. (three percent reservation)	No	0
	Total (%age)	11	8/11 (72.72%)

MOV- Q57to 62,65,66--(NHFDC office, Sec 17 and Annual Report Social Welfare Department)

-Q63,64—(Annual report of Social Welfare Department)

-Q67website of Urban Poverty Alleviation and livelihood Cell. Online at :mcchandigarh. gov.in/UPA.htm#link3.

Barrier free environment

Barrier free Environment includes independent movement of an individual with any kind of disability around the city without any problem and external support.

Prov./Q.no	Barrier free environment	Availability	Score
51(i)/68	All public buildings, modes of transportation, roads, and subways disabled friendly?	No	0
51(ii)/69	Use of sign languages at all public functions	No	0
51(iii)/70	Modification of curriculum of architects and civil engineers for constructing barrier free buildings.	Yes	1
51(iii)/71	In service trainings to the government architects and engineers	Yes	1
51(iv)/72	Full adoption of building byelaws for ensuring disabled friendly workplaces in public use.	Yes	1
51(v)/73	State transport Undertaking to ensure disabled friendly features in their vehicles.*	Yes	0.5
51(v)/74	Disabled friendly coaches, platforms and toilets.	No	0
51(vi)/75	Disabled friendly work place and security standards in public and private sector for their employees	No	0
51(vii)/76	Steps for disabled friendly IT environment**	No	0
51(viii)/77	Regular access auditing of the buildings	Yes	1
51(x)/78	Availability of public documents in Braille, large prints, tape services etc.***	Yes	0.5
	Total (11)	5.5/11= (50%)	

* low floor buses by Chandigarh Transport Undertaking; support PWDs other than wheelchair users.

*** State library sec 17 and Sec 34 has Braille and e-library for disabled but not all public documents available.

MOV -Q68,69,75,77—(observations and office of CPWD)

-Q70,71,72—Interview with Government architect and private Civil Engineer

- Q73,74—CTU office and Observation

- Q76-- Disability not mentioned in Information Technology and Electronics Policy, Chandigarh, 2013

-Q78—Department of Education and Interview with Librarian

Social security

Provision/ Q. no	Evaluation Parameter	Availability (yes/no)	Score obtained
34./79	Disability certificates issued within a month of applying.	Yes	1
35(i)/80	Unemployment allowance given to the registered unemployed disabled persons.	Yes	1
35(ii)/81	Any comprehensive social security plan available with UT admin, Chandigarh	Yes	1
35(iii)/82	Facilities in transportation for PWDs Concessional travel in CTU and Subsidy on petrol	Yes	1
35(iv)/83	Allotment of booths for supporting daily living	Yes	1
36. /84	Any support/legal guardianship scheme running in Chandigarh	Yes	1
38. /85	Information on disability being collected every five year	Yes	1
39. /86	Official websites accessible to visually impaired using screen reading technologies	No	0
52(iii)/87	All insurance agencies covering PWDs without exception	No	0

Promotion of NGOs

Provision/ Q. no.	Evaluation Parameter	Availability	Scores obtd.
37(i)/88	Is the directory of NGOs working on disability present?	Yes	1
37(iii)/89	Are the minimum standards, codes of conduct and ethics described, for NGOs working with PWD?	Yes	1
37(iv)/90.	If grants in aid and other kind of assistance are being provided to NGOs?	Yes	1

Women with disability

Provision/ Q.No.	Evaluation Parameter	Availability	Scores obtd.
29(i)/91	Special educational and vocational training available to disabled women?	No	0
29(ii)/92	Separate programmes for adoption of abandoned disabled women.	No	0
29(iii)/93	Projects available where representation of women with disability is at least 25% of total beneficiaries?	No	0
30./94	Separate short duration homes/ hostels available for working disabled /old women?	No	0
31./95	Financial support provided to mothers with disabilities to take care of their children	No	0
	Cumulative total (9+3+5=17)	7+3+0=10, 10/17=58.82%	

MOV:

-Q 79 to 85,88 to 90- (Department of Social Welfare).

-Q91 to 95- Annual report of Social welfare 2012-2013 did not mention special provisions about women with disabilities.

-Q86- observation, Q87—Interview with manager of a State Bank. (Bank do not cover PWD).

Research

The policy recognizes research for the holistic development of the differently able people. The city includes a large a number of research institutes like Post Graduate Institute of Medical Education and Research (PGIMER), Punjab University, National Institute of Technical Teachers Training and Research (NITTER), CSIO (Central Scientific Instrumental Organization) and Department of Science and Technology.

Provision/ Q.No.	Evaluation Parameters	Availability	Points obtained
53(i)/96.	Socio cultural aspects	Yes	1
53(ii)/97	Social indicators related to education of PWDs to improve programs	No	0
53(iii)/98	Statistics about employment status of disabled due to accidents and other disasters	No	0
53(iv)/99	Study of causes and level of incidence of disabilities	Partial (data collected on incidence only)	0.5
53(v)/100	Genetic research	Yes (GMCH)	1
53(vi)/101	Research on Adaptive technologies	Yes (CSIO/Nevdak)	1
	Science And Technology Department		
54(i)/102	Presence of Rehabilitation technology Center	No	0
54(ii)/103	Dedicated Budget	No	0
/104	Proposed/ working project	No	0
/105	Coordination with other centers	No	0
	Total (10)		3.5/10=35%

MOV:

-Q96 to 99-- Information not available anywhere on website of Chandigarh Administration and from the annual reports of Department of Statistics and Social welfare Department.

Q100- Website of GMCH sector 32.

Q101- Interview with the scientist working for disability in CSIO, Sector 31.

Q102 to105- Department of Science and Technology.

Sports and recreation and cultural activities

Policy includes provision for accessible recreational centers, hotels, sports auditoriums, malls etc to provide them social inclusion in the society.

Prov/Q.no	Evaluation Parameter	Availability	Score obtained
55(i)/106	Places for recreation, cultural activity, hotels, gyms auditoriums for PWDs	No	0
55(ii)/107	Travel agencies and voluntary organizations organizing recreational activities for PWDs.	No	0
55(iii)/108	Identifying sports talent among PWDs with the help of NGO.	No	0
55(iv)/109	Formation of sports organizations and cultural societies for PWDs.	No	0
55(v)/110	National award for excellence in sports for PWDs.	Yes	1
	Total		1/5 (20%)

MOV-Q106,107—Department of Tourism.

- Q108 to 110—District Sports Officer, Department of Sports, Sector 42.

In: Disability: International Aspects
Editors: Ariel Tenenbaum et al.
ISBN: 978-1-53617-886-9

Chapter 8

COMPLIANCE WITH SECTION 6 OF THE PERSONS WITH DISABILITY ACT 715: A CASE STUDY OF KUMASI POLYTECHNIC

Naomi Gyamfi*, Bsc, Msc Candidate and Akwasi Adjei Gyimah, Bsc, Msc Candidate
Centre for Disability and Rehabilitation Studies,
Department of Community Health,
School of Medical Sciences Kwame
Nkrumah University of Science and Technology,
Kumasi, Ghana

ABSTRACT

Section 6 of the Persons with Disability Act 715 of Ghana requires that all public places must be made accessible to persons with disabilities to ensure their inclusion in society. However, it is uncertain how this Act is

* Corresponding Author: Gyamfi N, a post-graduate student at Centre for Disability and Rehabilitation Studies, Department of Community Health, School of Medical Sciences, Kwame Nkrumah University of Science and Technology. E-mail: naomi.gyamfi@yahoo.com.

being complied with by public institutions. This study sought to examine the accessibility of Kumasi Polytechnic (now known as Kumasi Technical University), a tertiary institution in Ghana, to students with physical disabilities. The study employed qualitative method using in-depth interview to gather information from 22 participants purposively selected. Findings from the study showed that physical environment of the school, such as lecture halls, halls of residence, and compound were not disability-friendly, and some students with physical disabilities had to rely on their friends to access the buildings or reallocate their classes. Also, most of the participants were not well-informed and knowledgeable about the Persons with Disability Act, and did not make efforts to demand for their rights. It is recommended that there should be a strong public education on the Persons with Disability Act so that people will be abreast with its content.

INTRODUCTION

Access to education is a fundamental human right to every child and this right is supported by various international legislations and conventions, and national constitutions. The Salamanca Framework for Action is a typical example of international efforts to increase access to education for all children, young people and adults within the regular education system (1). However, studies have shown that many children with disabilities have no or lower educational attainment than other children. They are also more likely to be enrolled in school late and leave earlier with fewer qualifications than other children (2, 3). Negative teacher attitude, inaccessible environment and rigid curriculum are some of the factors accounting for the low education of children with disabilities (4, 5). For persons with physical disabilities, inaccessible physical environment, such as, poorly designed ramps, steep and poorly designed staircases, non-availability of lifts, unpaved access route, and narrow entry doors are major barrier that hinder their enrolment and participation (6-8). Those who get enrolled, face numerous barriers and are often supported by their peers or/ and arrange for relocation of their classes, for example, on the ground floor (6, 9). However, these measures do not often tackle the root cause of the barriers and as a result, have not completely increased the participation of such children in school activities (6).

Legal framework

This study is influenced by provisions in the United Nations Convention on the Rights of Persons with Disabilities (CRPDs) and Persons with Disability Act 715 of Ghana (10).

Convention on the Rights of Persons with Disabilities

Inclusion of persons with disabilities in education has been supported globally by anti-discriminatory legislations. These legislations include the convention on the right of persons with disabilities (CRPDs). The CRPD is the first broad international treaty that specifically protects the human rights of persons with disabilities. The main purpose of the CRPDs is to promote, protect and ensure the full and equal enjoyment of all human rights and fundamental freedoms on all persons with disabilities, and to promote respect for their inherent dignity. Article 24 and 4 enjoins signatory countries to make education inclusive for PWDs at all levels and to ensure ease access.

Persons with Disability Act

The Persons with Disability Act 715 of Ghana has provisions in Section 6 which states that, "The owner or occupier of a place to which the public has access shall provide facilities that make the place accessible to and available for use by a person with disability"(10). This means that all barriers in public places, including educational institutions, should be removed to make them accessible to persons with disabilities.

Since the enactment of the Persons with Disability Act 715, a lot of activities have taken place to ensure compliance with its provision. However, there are many obstacles to the implementation of the Act. One of major obstacles is that many buildings were designed with no accessibility feature and it will be difficult to redesign most of these buildings to make them accessible. This presents a serious conundrum for authorities in educational institutions, who are obliged to admit all persons who apply to their institution. It is uncertain if educational institutions are aware of provisions in the Act and if they are taking steps to respond to the needs of students with physical disabilities. This study investigated the inclusion of students with physical disabilities in a tertiary education setting in Ghana by using Kumasi Polytechnic (now known as Kumasi Technical University) as a case.

OUR STUDY

Kumasi Polytechnic is one of the 10 polytechnics in Ghana located in Kumasi, the capital city of the Ashanti Region of Ghana. The school has a population of 4,722 students at the time of the study. The only students with disabilities admitted in the institution were those with physical disabilities, but there were no data on the number of these students in the institution. In terms of accessibility, most of the buildings in the institution were not accessible; most of the buildings were storey and so most of the offices, lecture halls, and halls of residence were located upstairs, that is, on the first, second, third and fourth floors. Even though the school is structurally storey, only the administration building has an elevator at the time of the study. There were also very few ramps in the school, as a result, many entrances to the rooms and office were not accessible to wheelchair users.

The study used a purposive sampling to enroll twenty-two participants. The participants consisted of ten students with physical disabilities, three students without disabilities, four administrators, and two heads of departments, three lecturers and one lift operator. Students without disabilities were included in the study because a preliminary study in the institution indicated that some of the staff encouraged these students to help their colleagues with disabilities. These students were friends of the students with physical disabilities interviewed.

A semi-structured interview guide was used for the study. The interview guide covered the demographic characteristics of participants, their level of awareness of the Persons with Disability Act, 715, the extent to which the school was complying with Section 6 of the Persons with Disability Act, 715, and the inclusion of students with physical disabilities in the school's activities. Following the consent of the participants, the interviews were recorded using audio-tapes. The study was conducted within four months.

The Committee on Human Research and Publication Ethics at the Kwame Nkrumah University of Science and Technology gave Consent for the study to be conducted. Also, the participants' consent was sought before they participated in the study. In addition, participants were assured that any information provided would remain secret; names and identity of participants were not revealed in this study. Lastly, participation was voluntary and participants were informed that they had the right to withdraw from the study at any point.

Ghana has 10 polytechnics located in the various regions. However, the study was limited to only Kumasi Polytechnic. Also, the study was limited to only students with physical disabilities and some friends of these students. These are shortcomings of the study that will make generalizing the findings to other institutions difficult. . Therefore it is recommended that future studies should include other institutions to provide comprehensive data on the situation in other institutions.

The recorded data from the interview were transcribed verbatim by the researcher. The researcher read through the transcripts several times to identify common themes that were related to the research objectives. Based on the objectives of the study, a coding system using colors was developed. Four colors, red, yellow, green and blue representing each of the four research questions were used to highlight the participants' responses that are consistent with each research question. All the responses related to research objective one were highlighted red, blue for objective two, yellow for objective three and green for objective four. Based on the colours, similar themes were grouped together to form the main themes of the study.

FINDINGS

Out of the total participants, 68% were males and half of the participants were within the age range of 21 to 29 years. In terms of marital status, more than half (59%) were single, with the remaining (41%) being married. The most represented students in the study were those in level three hundred, with staff being 45%. For the summary of the demographic characteristics, see Table (1).

Table 1. Demographic distribution of participants

Variable	Number of participants	Percentages (%)
Sex		
Male	15	68
Female	7	32
Total	22	100
Age		
16-20	3	14
21-29	12	55
30-39	5	23
40 and above	2	9
total	22	100
Marital status		
Married	9	41
Single	13	59
Total	22	100
Level of students		
hundred	1	5
Three hundred	5	23
Four hundred	6	27
None(staff)	10	45
Total	22	100

Awareness of the Persons with Disability Act 715

About 60% of the participants, including students with physical disabilities, said they were not aware of the Persons with Disability Act. The lack of awareness could be attributed to a general lack of interest in disability issues among the participants. One student with disability, for example, said "I am not aware of the Act, maybe because I don't join any disability association." Similarly, one lecturer indicated that "I don't really follow issues on disability. What I know is that everybody irrespective of the person's status, gender, race, age, educational background has his/her own rights and those rights must not be infringed upon. But for the Persons with Disability Act, I don't think I know about it." The findings also revealed that the few participants who were aware of the Act did not know its content. For example, while a student said that "I have heard about the Act but I don't know all the provisions in it" an administrator said "I know something like that exists. I know that is meant to ensure the enjoyment of human rights by persons with disabilities. I have a general knowledge about the Act but I don't know the provisions in it. I think it would have been better to know something small for this interview." Knowledge of the Act and its content is vital for its compliance by the school authorities, and for the students to demand implementation. The lack of awareness by both students and the school administrators implies that provisions in the Act. Including Section 6 are unlikely to be implemented.

Accessibility of the institution

Responses from the participants revealed that the physical environment of the institution was not accessible to students with physical disabilities. All the participants agreed that apart from their library which was situated within the administration block (the administration block is the only building with an elevator), all other facilities did not have elevators. A student said As a matter of fact, Kumasi Polytechnic is not accessible to students with disabilities. Buildings are not accessible; environment is not accessible, especially to wheel chair users. The rough nature of our environment does not permit easy movement of students in wheelchairs. Also, lack of ramps in most of the entrances and offices make movement on campus very difficult." A lecturer added that "our lecture halls do not have elevators. But classes which include students with physical disabilities are held on the ground floor. We make arrangements with students to select classes they can easily access. There are only few instances where we take classes on top of the buildings." One head of department also said "As you can see, our leaders did not consider the needs of persons with disabilities when they were putting up this institution. All our buildings are storey, without elevators except our administration which was currently put up." Finally the lift operator added that "It is pathetic that almost all the buildings here are multiple floors, but our government did not consider a population of human being who will have difficulties in climbing. I am the regulator of this elevator and this is the only elevator we have in this school. They said I shouldn't allow students to use but for students with physical disabilities I consider them because they can use this to get to the school's library so I allow them to use." It could be seen from the above that students with physical disabilities were encountering several barriers. The attempts being made to address these problems are unplanned and they were temporarily and not being done as required by the Act.

Readiness to implement the Act

The implementation of Section 6 of the Act will require retrofitting of buildings and changing practices in the institution to suit the needs of students with physical disabilities so that they can participate fully in activities in the institution. It generally emerged that the institution has not yet responded to the provisions in the section 6 of the Act. However, the views of the participants were split among those who perceived internal arrangement to support students with physical disabilities and those who perceived these arrangements as only made to respond to the needs of lecturers with disabilities. The second head of department said "I am not sure of restructuring of facilities in in the school with the aim of making it accessible to students with physical disabilities. What I know is that their classes are normally on the ground floor. What we do is that we ask the class prefect to submit programmes that have persons with physical disabilities in it… and when we get to know the programmes or the level, we intend to bring their classes to the ground floor that is what we do for them to access lectures but for other events I don't know." One student added that "They are not implementing any Act. You can ask my friends most of our classes are on the last floor of our building. I struggle to get there. I once fought with my head... I went to him to tell him that all my classes are on the last floor so he should help and bring some to the ground floor to make things easier for me. He told me that he was not the one who did the allocation of classes, and that it came from the top management so he could not do anything about it. Meanwhile I know a lecturer with disabilities who has all his classes on the ground floor. So why should they have compassion on the lecturer and neglect we the students"

However, Participants explained that students with physical disabilities were included in most social activities though the physical environment seems not accessible. These activities were mostly visiting cinema halls, sporting, and leadership positions among students. This was realized when the needs of students with physical disabilities are considered in planning these social events and activities. One said: Students with disabilities are included in all social activities. Some competes for leadership positions, they are able to join lectures, and their needs are considered when planning any social events on campus. Even in difficult times, we advise their colleagues without disabilities to help them" (Head of a Department. A student added that "We are not excluded from social activities in the school. For example, when it comes to leadership position every student can apply whether able or disabled and when you qualify to be in that position it will be given to you. Our course mates and friends welcome us in all social activities like sporting activities. They don't discriminate against us; they sometimes even help us with carrying our wheel chairs. So for social activities, I don't think we are excluded but the point is, sometimes we don't feel like joining those events" Another said "We do everything together with our peers with physical disabilities. You see, one of them is my roommates and we do everything together. We don't fear them because we know they are like us, just that they are unfortunate to suffer those sicknesses. We sometimes help them in carrying their clutches and wheel chairs" (student without disabilities).

Participants further explained that students with physical disabilities do not face discrimination and many of them receive support from their peers without disabilities. Students with disabilities for instance felt that they were being treated fairly by their peers and had good relationship with them. One student with disability, for example, indicated that "we don't face discrimination from lecturers and students without disabilities. No verbal abuse from workers unlike other institutions but our problem is on the inaccessibility of the facilities."

In summary, although there seemed to be lack of awareness of provisions in the Disability Act and the school environment was inaccessible, excluding many students with physically disabilities from mainstream activities, there seemed to be efforts to include them in schools activities.

Discussion

The study investigated the compliance of Kumasi Polytechnic with the Persons with Disability Act 715. It specifically examined the extent to which the school's activities and structures respond to Section 6 of the Act. The focus of the study was school administrators, Lecturers and students with physical disabilities and their friends.

The study found that most of the participants in the study were not privy to the content of the Persons with Disability Act 715 implying that they were also unaware of the rights of the students under the Act. This lack of awareness is probably the cause of non-compliance with the Act as the findings of the study indicated. The findings indicating that the school environment was not accessible are therefore expected and consistent with some studies which have found that inaccessible school environment was a general problem in many educational institutions in Ghana (6-8). Also, studies elsewhere found that students with physical disabilities were unable to participate in school activities due to inaccessible physical environment (4, 5).

Even though some of the students received support from their colleagues, which suggests a positive attitude towards students with physical disabilities, dependence on their peers is not the best solution. This support is unreliable which would not give students with physical disabilities the level of independence they need; they would have to depend on the generosity of their peers. However, this may be the best alternative for these students because it is unlikely the environment of the school will be made accessible in the near future due to the architectural and financial constraints and lack of a clear institutional plan as well as pragmatic actions by various students' bodies, disability groups and government to ensure the implementation of the Persons with Disability Act, 715.

The positive attitude towards students with physical disabilities suggests shifted of attitude to the positive side and this may have been influenced by increased in advocacy on disability issues or constant interaction between students with physical disabilities and their peers without disabilities. It could also be due to the level of education of the residence in the institution. Recall that the study was conducted in an academic institution, and thus, even though many of residence in the institution were unaware of the provisions in the Act, their educational attainment might have caused them to think and behave positively towards persons with disabilities.

Few studies have focused on accessibility issues in educational institutions in Ghana. Findings from these studies indicated that the physical environment in many educational institutions in Ghana were not accessible to persons with disabilities because they were not originally designed to accommodate persons with disabilities (6-8). This implies that a lot of resources will be needed to retrofit our educational institutions to make them accessible in order to enhance the implementation of inclusive education policy currently being implemented.

This study has several implications for policy-making on the implementation of provisions in the Persons with Disability Act 715. Since one of the findings is that people were not abreast with provisions in the Act, there should be intensive public education on the Act in the media such as television stations, information centers, and radio station to create awareness. Also, the World Disability Day could be used as an opportunity for persons with disabilities and their advocates to educate the general public on disability issues, including provisions in the Act.

While education is important to change perceptions about disability, education alone cannot cause the needed change without enforcing laws prohibiting discrimination against persons with disabilities. Existing laws prohibiting unfair treatment against persons with disabilities should therefore be enforced.

Additionally, since public educational institutions rely on the central government for their funds, it means these institutions can do little about making their environment accessible without government support. Government should therefore provide adequate resources to the institutions to enable them modify their environment. Although this will be difficult for the government due to the current state of Ghana's economy, cost should not be used as an excuse to deny students with physical disabilities their right to use facilities in these institutions. Since most of the public institutions generate income internally, some of the funds generated could be used to support government's efforts at increasing access to higher education for students with disabilities.

It is important, however, to note that even if service providers are willing to make their environment accessible this cannot be done without accessibility guidelines to guide them. The National Council on Persons with Disability and the Ghana Standard Board should therefore fast-track the development of the National Accessible Guidelines to guide the implementation of accessibility provisions in the Act.

ACKNOWLEDGMENTS

The author acknowledges the staff and students at Kumasi Technical University for their immense contributions towards the successful completion of this study.

REFERENCES

[1] The United Nations Educational Scientific and Cultural Organization [UNESCO]. The Dakar Framework for Action. Dakar, Senegal/Paris: United Nations, 2000.

[2] World Health Organization. World report on disability. Geneva: World Health Organization, 2011.

[3] Ametepee LK, Anastasiou D. Special and inclusive education in Ghana: Status and progress, challenges and implications. Int J Educ Dev 2015;41:143-52.

[4] Garriott PP, Miller M, Snyder L. Preservice teachers' beliefs about inclusive education: What should teacher educators know?. Action Teacher Educ. 2003;25(1):48-54.

[5] Rakap, S.Teacher's attitudes towards inclusion/integration in Turkey. Paper presented at the 2nd International Conference on Special Education. Turkey: Marmaris, Mugla, 2008.

[6] Danso AK, Owusu-Ansah FE, Alorwu D. Designed to deter: barriers to facilities at secondary schools in Ghana: original research. Afr J Disabil 2012;1(1):1-9.

[7] Mprah WK, Amponteng M, Owusu I. Barriers to inclusion of children with disabilities in inclusive schools in Ghana. J Disabil Stud 2015;1(1):15-22.

[8] Opoku MP, Badu E, Amponteng M, Agyei-Okyere E. Inclusive Education at the crossroads in Ashanti and BrongAhafo regions in Ghana: Target not achievable by 2015. Disabil CBR Inclusive Dev 2015;26(1):63-78.

[9] Morley L, Croft A. Agency and advocacy: Disabled students in higher education in Ghana and Tanzania. Res Comparat Int Educ 2011;6(4):383-99.

[10] Persons with Disability Act. 175th Act of the Parliament of the Republic of Ghana. Accra: Ghana Publishing, 2006.

In: Disability: International Aspects
Editors: Ariel Tenenbaum et al.
ISBN: 978-1-53617-886-9

Chapter 9

NARRATIVE COMPREHENSION AND EXPRESSION IN MALAYALAM SPEAKING CHILDREN WITH CEREBRAL PALSY

Dayana Devassy[1], MASLP, Sunila John[2], PhD, Damodar K Veena[2,*], PhD and Bellur Rajashekhar[2], PhD

[1]Amrita Institute of Medical Science and Research Centre, Kochi
[2]Department of Speech and Hearing, School of Allied Health Sciences, Manipal University, Manipal, Karnataka, India

ABSTRACT

Narratives is a form of discourse, which includes use of a series of sentences to describe an event. In the present study, narrative skills were investigated in 20 children with cerebral palsy (CP) and 20 typically developing (TD) children between 5 to 13 years. Both narrative

* Corresponding Author: Associate professor, Damodar K Veena, Department of Speech and Hearing, School of Allied Health Sciences, Manipal University, Karnataka, India.
E-mail: r.veena@manipal.edu.

comprehension and narrative expression (macro-structural and microstructural analysis) were explored. Narrative macrostructure analysis focused on scores obtained for story content, event, grammar and story. Narrative microstructure analysis included type-token ratio (TTR), mean length of utterance (MLU) and number of sentences (NS). The study findings revealed a reduced performance in children with CP in all the measures with statistically significant difference for the tasks of narrative comprehension and TTR. The study indicates the relevance of using narrative analysis along with the standard test protocol for language assessment in children with CP.

INTRODUCTION

Discourse is one aspect of pragmatics, which has been used to refer to conversations or sentence strings in monologue. It is studied at two levels: microstructural and macro-structural. The local or microstructure level pertains to connections between sentences and can be studied with sentence pattern. Broad themes and structural scheme appears at the global or macro-structural level (1). Among the different types of discourse identified, narratives are a form of discourse, which includes use of a series of sentences to describe an event. Narrative discourse can be viewed as a quasi-naturalistic measure to explore the language ability in children. It is an orderly account of real or imagined events. A very simple narrative contains few utterances about the common theme. More complex narrative may contain descriptions about multiple people who engage in goal-directed actions.

Children engage in narratives almost from the time they begin talking. Soon thereafter, they begin to understand the narrative speech of others and start to conceptualize and tell their own stories. Narrative skills undergo many changes during the elementary school years. At the macrostructure level, according to Stein and Glenn (2), story grammar system appears to capture many of the developmental changes in spontaneously generated stories and in story retelling between 5 and 12 years olds. The oral narratives of most children of kindergarten contain basic episode (an initiating event, goal directed actions and a consequence), but not being consistent across story telling context. Older children tend to include more story preposition in their oral narrative than younger children. Children in third through fifth grade are better than kindergartners at generating stories that contain multiple goal based actions with one or more obstacle, elaborated endings, internal response, plans, reactions and multiple conjoined or embedded episode. Children between the ages of 5 and 6 years can be expected to provide some setting information, basic information about the characters, basic temporal markers such as "and then," and some character dialogue. Children's between the ages of 10 and 11 years include multiple mental verbs, temporal adverbs, and casual adverbs in their stories.

Narration is an amalgamation of one's ability to use the syntactic, semantic and other component of language in socially relevant manner. Narrative has been reported to be a valid predictor of deficits in language and literacy skills (3). Moreover, it is useful for differentiating various subgroups in children with communication difficulties (4). It has gained importance in clinical evaluation in many childhood language disorders including autism, intellectual disability, William syndrome, Down's syndrome, specific language impairment and learning disability (5-7).

Though many studies have been done on discourse, very few studies have been reported in children with cerebral palsy (CP). It refers to a group of disorders affecting development of movement and posture, causing activity limitation due to disturbances in brain development (8). The incidence of CP is 1.5 to 3.5 per 1,000 births in India (9). In general, studies among English speaking children with CP reveal presence of communication impairment with poor performance in linguistic aspects as compared to typically developing children (TD) (10, 11).

Feldman et al. (12) reported lack of significant difference between CP associated with perinatal injury to the periventricular white matter of the brain and children with no brain injury on discourse measures of type-token ratio per minute, number of grammatical morpheme, mean length of utterance and number of utterance per minute. In the Scott and Hidecker (13) study, narrative performance of children with CP was compared across different communication partners (familiar vs unfamiliar partner).

The results revealed that the mean length of utterance per language sample, speech comprehensibility and type-token were similar across the partners. Contrary to this finding, Hemphill et al. and Holck et a. (5, 14) reported delayed narrative ability in children with CP. In Holck et al. study, no significant difference in terms of information and mean length of utterance, topic maintenance, explicitness, event sequencing, reference and fluency were noted between children with CP and control group. However, a significant difference was reported in terms of use of conjunctions and subordinate clauses. A positive correlation between narrative ability on story re-telling tasks and receptive and expressive language skills are also reported in literature (15). In Indian context, there is a dearth of information on performance of children with CP on narrative discourse. Chengappa, Bhat and Iyer (16) reported reduced mean length of utterance among Kannada speaking children with CP. In terms of syntactic complexity, compound verbs and inflections were limited in children with CP. Children produced nouns more frequently as compared to verbs and pronouns. The authors attributed the poor performance of children with CP as compared to normal to articulatory insufficiency. The study findings indicated that age does not emerge as a definite variable of language skills in CP but is influenced by severity with deviance in speech production.

The present study evaluated the extent to which measure narrative ability is impaired in children with CP as compared to typically developing children in Malayalam language. Malayalam (belonging to Dravidian family of languages) is the native language spoken in the state of Kerala, a South Indian state and is considered as one of the 22 official languages in India. Presence of a significant difference in the narrative ability among the two groups indicates the efficacy of using narrative discourse as a clinical tool for language assessment and later for treatment aspects for children with cerebral palsy. The objectives of the present study were comparison of narrative ability in terms of narrative comprehension and narrative expression in children with CP. It was hypothesized that, children with CP performs poorer than typically developing children in narrative discourse.

OUR STUDY

A total of 40 children with Malayalam as their native language participated in the study. The TD children and children with CP formed the two groups of participants. Children with CP group consisted of verbal children (n = 20) with age adequate language skills; intelligence quotient greater than 70 and spastic diplegic CP type. Children with TD (n = 20) group consisted of language age matched, typically developing children, attending normal school. All the children in Group 1 were provided the impression of childhood dysarthria by Speech Language Pathologist and Group 2 comprised of children with clinically normal speech and language skills.

Table 1. Demographic and clinical data of children with (CP) and Typically Developing (TD)

Characteristics	CP (n = 20)	TD (n = 20)
Age	9 years 1 months	8 years 6 months
Boys	9	12
Girls	11	8
IQ score	*87.45 (Mean)*	Not tested
Type of cerebral palsy	*Spastic diplegia*	Not applicable
Speech diagnosis	*Childhood dysarthria with functionally adequate language skills*	Clinically normal speech and language skills
Schooling	*Attending normal school/special school*	*Attending normal school*

The narrative was elicited from all the participants in Malayalam language for two task namely narrative comprehension and narrative expression. For narrative comprehension task, a short story consisting of 6 sequenced black and white pictures of "thirsty crow" was used. The child was instructed that "I am going to tell you a story that goes with the picture that you see here. I want you to listen carefully, is it clear. Later I am going to ask you few questions about the story, Are you ready?" The story was narrated by the investigator and following the story narration nine comprehensive questions were asked based on the story. After each question the answers were noted down by the investigator by a tick mark indicating the correct response and cross indicating the incorrect response.

For narrative expression task a different story picture cards (six sequenced black and white picture cards) of “hare and the tortoise” were used for story retelling task. For story retelling task, the children were shown a six sequence picture cards and instructed “Now I will tell you a story that goes with the six-sequence picture card. After I complete I want you to retell the story. Make your story as long as you can.” If the subject had difficulty getting started, the investigator asked the subject, “What can you see in the picture? Name the animals that you see in the picture?” The story retelling was audio recorded using a digital voice recorder and was stored for further analysis.

ANALYSIS

The analysis included both narrative comprehension and narrative expression. In comprehension task, a total of nine comprehension questions were asked. Each comprehension question carried one mark respectively. Thus, a maximum score of 9-point and a minimum score of 0-point can be scored by the participants. In narrative expression task, the recorded speech samples were transcribed by the investigator. Incomplete and unintelligible utterances were not included for analysis. The transcribed speech samples were further analysed for microstructure and macro-structural aspects of narratives.

Narrative macrostructure analysis included Test for Narrative Language (TNL) (17) score, comprising of sum of the scores obtained for story content, event, grammar and story. Based on TNL scoring, a maximum of 18 score was given for the story content, if the child was able to provide all the information about the story character, conversation, setting, movement, reaction or felling and moral or ending. Event represents temporal relationship between events (e.g., uses “and” or “then,” uses one or more adverbial phrases or clauses). Grammar represents the use of grammatically correct sentence (e.g., listen for grammatical errors such as "tortoise comes first"). Scoring for the story was based on the investigator's overall judgement about the coherence of the story, that is how each statement (subject- verb-object unit) relates to the story as a whole (e.g., a scoring of 0 indicates two or more statements do not make sense with reference to the entire story). A maximum of 4-point and a minimum of 0-point were scored participants for the event, grammar and story. The total score (maximum score of 30-point) for the narrative macrostructure analysis was computed by the sum of story content, story, event, grammar and story.

Narrative microstructure analysis included type-token ratio (TTR), mean length of utterance (MLU) and number of sentences (NS). TTR is calculated in morphemes by dividing the total number of morphemes divided by the total number of utterances (For example in the sentence "/amma oru mutham thannu/." the MLU is 4). Type token ratio is the ratio of the number of different words used in a sample to the number of total words used in the sample. For example, in a paragraph containing 245 tokens (total words), but only 132 types (different words), the type-token ratio was 53.88 (132/245 × 100). Analysis also included the calculation of number of sentences in the speech sample.

Statistical analysis was done using Independent t test was used to find whether there is a statistically significant difference between the means in two unrelated groups. The p value was set at 0.05 levels of significance. All the statistical analysis was done using Statistical Package for Social Science, Chicago Inc. version-15.

FINDINGS

Narrative ability in children with CP was assessed in terms of narrative comprehension and narrative expression. Overall, performance on narrative comprehension was found to be better than narrative expression.

Table 2. Comparison of narrative skills between children with CP and TD children

	CP Mean(SD)	TD Mean (SD)	p-value
Narrative comprehension	7.15(2.34)	8.9(0.3)	0.001*
Narrative expression			
TNL score	17.75(7.37)	19.35(3.10)	0.47
MLU	4.85(2.12)	5.23(0.88)	0.47
TTR (median, Interquartile range)	0.7,0.1	0.7, 0.1	0.04*
Number of sentences	7.15(2.39)	8.65(2.43)	0.06

Note: * indicate significant difference at p value < 0.05 level.

As indicated in Table 2, in terms of narrative comprehension task, the children with CP obtained a mean score of 7.15 (*SD* = 2.34) while the TD children had a mean of 8.9 (*SD* = 0.3) which was statistically significant.

In narrative expression macrostructure analysis that is the TNL score, children with CP scored a mean of 17.75 (*SD* = 7.37) and TD children had a mean of 19.4(*SD* = 2.93). In narrative expression microstructure analysis with respect to MLU, children with CP had a mean of 4.85(*SD* = 2.11) and TD children had a mean of 5.25(*SD* = 0.87). With respect to TTR, the median value for children with CP is 0.7 (Interquartile range = 0.1) and TD children had a mean of 0.73 (*SD* = 0.07). And with respect to NS, children with CP had a mean of 7.15 (*SD* = 2.39) and TD children had a mean of 8.65(*SD* = 2.43). Among, the various microstructural outcome measures, only the TTR scores were statistically significant as indicated in Table 2.

DISCUSSION

In the present study, it was observed that children with CP performed poorly on narrative comprehension and narrative expression as compared to TD. Similar findings of reduced narrative ability have been reported (5, 18). Holck et al. (18) suggested that narrative ability in children with CP were delayed rather than deviant. In the present study despite children with

CP having age adequate language skills, deficits in narrative skills were observed. This presence of narrative deficits indicates that narrative evaluation in terms of comprehension and expression needs to be part of routine language evaluation in children with CP, which may be otherwise missed if we depend purely on just a standard language test.

In terms of narrative comprehension, the TD showed better performance compared to children with CP. Most of the children in TD group showed superior performance with a score of 8-point or 9-point (on a maximum score of 9-point) whereas scores of children with CP ranged from 1-point to 9-point. It was also noted that with increase in age, narrative performance showed improved performance. Most of the children (n = 11) with CP above the age of 9-years-old could score more than 8-points whereas children above age of 5-years-old scored less than 6-points. This can be attributed to their deficit in area of executive functioning including sustained attention and use of efficient and organized strategies for learning (19). Moreover, 16 out of 20 children with CP were not able to answer for the ninth question regarding the behavior of the crow (the expected answer being "crow is intelligent"), but they could answer for the remaining questions. This difficulty in narrative comprehension seen in children with CP can be because of their difficulty with inferential ability. Similar finding in literature is reported by Holck et al. (18), where they reported that inferential comprehension related to language comprehension is affected in children with CP.

The present study also compared the narrative expression on story in terms of story retelling task. The analysis included the macro-structural (Test of Narrative Language score) and micro-structural level (Mean Length of Utterance (MLU), Type Token Ratio (TTR) and number of sentences used). Story retelling task was used rather than story generation, as story generation is considered to be more challenging than story retelling. According to Leinonen et al. (20) story retelling emerges from child itself without external input. Boudreau (21) also pointed out that story retelling is less demanding and this is more appropriate for preschool-aged children. According to Hudson and Shapiro (22), story retelling is advantageous, as the evaluator is familiar with the content of the story.

In macro-analysis of narrative expression using Test of Narrative Language (TNL) (include four components of narrative expression assessment: story content, story, event and grammar), the present study finding showed as inferior performance of children with CP as compared to TD children. During the story narration, children with CP showed preservative errors such as repeating the phrase "it's a rabbit" for all the picture cards. In the narrative samples of children with CP (n = 8) there has been abrupt shift between the events (e.g., the child says "Once there lived a hare and a tortoise. When they kept race, tortoise came first"), as they tried to describe the picture rather than formulating a creative story out of the picture. A very few (n = 4) children with CP were able to mentioned the conversation and moral of the story. Their inability to make inferential statements can be because of the underlying lesion present in children with CP, resulting in wide array of cognitive impairment. According to Luciana (23) due to the lesion in white matter tracts the children with CP are likely to exhibit lower efficiency of information processing. Their inability to retell the complete and elaborate stories also could be due to their problem with short- term memory (24). Norbury and Bishop (25) found similar results in their study and reported that children with CP used causal conjunctions significantly less than TD group. These difficulties result in increased risk of developing Specific language impairment or Learning disability in children with CP. Similar to Straub and Obrzut (24) findings, in the current study children with CP showed inability to frame an integrated story line, elaboration, humour, surprise or other creative element. However, the children with above average IQ (>117) could formulate a complete story with more creativity, humor and surprise.

Among micro analysis component considered for analysis of narrative expression was Mean Length of Utterance (MLU), Type Token Ratio (TTR) and Number of Sentence (NS). MLU is considered as a measure of the syntactic complexity of the language. According to Brown's stage (26) of MLU, children in CP and TD group fall within the stage five (co-ordination; MLU = 3.75- 4.25 with average of four morphemes; the child may use more connectors and more functions as "Mom is in the car"). Chengappa et al. (16) reported an MLU of 2.69 for children with CP and 4.14 for TD group in Kannada between the age ranges of 4-11 years. In the present study MLU was reduced in children with CP as compared to TD group, although there was no significant difference was found. MLU has been found to be sensitive to several intra individual and extra individual differences, as described by various researchers. Some of the intra individual variables include interest in the topic, and familiarity with the topic. The possible reasons for a lower performance of children with CP compared to TD could be because of the difference in location of elicitation of language sample, interest in the topic, familiarity with the topic. As in the present study, language samples of children with CP were collected from clinical setting and those of TD children from their home. Similar findings have been reported in the literature (27). They reported a better MLU for home sample as compared to clinical setting in three to five-year-old children.

In terms of TTR, there was a significant difference in children with CP compared to the TD group. TTR indicates the linguistic complexity of the production. A lower score would indicate the use of simple language in the narrative sample. A higher score indicates greater linguistic complexity. This outcome supports the study by Templin (28) who examined the 50-utterance narrative sample of 480 children between the ages of 3 - 8 year. Templin's study reported a TTR of approximately 0.50 across the age span and did not vary by gender or socioeconomic status. In the present study the TTR obtained for both the group were 0.7 (median) an average of 50 utterances sample were collected for both the age group. The better performance of TTR in Group 2 compared to Group 1 could be because of the difference in narrative sample size. As the number of utterance in a sample increases, words tend to be repeated and hence the TTR might decrease (29). Contrary to this study, Richard (30) reported that TTR is not a valid measure to measure lexical diversity as it is influenced by the sample size. In the present study children with CP used considerably less number of types (different words) but more number of tokens (total words) as compared to the TD group. There was increased number of preservative errors and repetition of sentences and words (during the attempts of self-correction) in the narrative sample of children with CP compared to TD group. This could have resulted in lower performance of this group as compared to TD group.

In terms of number of sentences, the study outcome indicates that there was no significant difference among the two groups, which could be attributed to the participant selection criteria of age adequate language skills. However, the total number of sentences in children with CP group was less compared to TD children. This difference could be because of their difficulty with short term memory (STM) and language processing. As reported by various investigators (31, 32), short term memory skills have been related to children's sentence recall. And since the STM and language processing is affected in children with CP, they might have difficulty in retelling the story.

Limitations

There are certain limitations that needs to be addressed in future research. In the present study, ascertaining pattern of changes in discourse among different age groups has not been measured as a wide age range was selected. Similarly, detailed narrative analysis measures like, counting T-units and subordinate clauses were not included which could have provided a better understanding of narrative performance in children with CP.

Conclusion

To conclude, the overall performance in narrative tasks was poorer in children with CP as compared to TD children. An understanding of the precise nature of the discourse would enable better understanding of discourse characteristics in children with CP and TD children. Studying discourse in normal individuals could provide a baseline to assist in the evaluation, a better method of evaluation, clinical data to compare with the language disorder population and development of assessment tool. It also helps in devising experimental therapy of for children with CP depending on deficit in discourse. This study has important application for assessment and intervention of children with CP. Besides assessing the semantic and syntactic aspects of language, narrative analysis also explores aspects of discourse that are not usually accessible with standard language test.

REFERENCES

[1] Heilmann J, Miller JF, Nockerts A, Dunaway C. Properties of the narrative scoring scheme using narrative retells in young school-age children. Am J Speech Lang Pathol 2010;19(2):154-66.

[2] Stein NL, Glenn CG. An analysis of story comprehension in elementary children, vol 2. Norwood, NJ: Ablex, 1979.

[3] Stothard SE, Snowling MJ, Bishop DV, Chipchase BB, Kaplan CA. Language-impaired preschoolers: A follow-up into adolescence. J Speech Lang Hear Res 1998;41(2):407-18.

[4] Botting N. Narrative as a tool for the assessment of linguistic and pragmatic impairments. Child Lang Teach Ther 2002;18(1):1-21.

[5] Holck P, Sandberg AD, Nettelbladt U. Narrative ability in children with cerebral palsy. Res Dev Disabil 2011;32(1):262-70.

[6] Losh M, Capps L. Narrative ability in high-functioning children with autism or Asperger's syndrome. J Autism Dev Disord 2003;33(3):239-51.

[7] Bliss LS, McCabe A, Miranda AE. Narrative assessment profile: Discourse analysis for school-age children. J Commun Disord 1998;31(4):347-63.

[8] Bax M, Goldstein M, Rosenbaum P, Leviton A, Paneth N, Dan B, et al. Proposed definition and classification of cerebral palsy, April 2005. Dev Med Child Neurol 2005;47(8):571-6.

[9] Srivastava VK, Laisram N, Srivastava RK. Cerebral palsy. Indian J Pediatrics 1992;29:993-6.

[10] Hanzlik JR, Stevenson MB. Interaction of mothers with their infants who are mentally retarded, retarded with cerebral palsy, or nonretarded. Am J Ment Defic 1986;90(5):513-20.

[11] Pennington L, Goldbart J, Marshall J. Interaction training for conversational partners of children with cerebral palsy: A systematic review. Int J Lang Commun Disord 2004;39(2):151-70.

[12] Feldman HM, Janosky JE, Scher MS, Wareham NL. Language abilities following prematurity, periventricular brain injury, and cerebral palsy. J Commun Disord 1994;27(2):71-90.

[13] Scott M, Hidecker MJC. Communication performance of children with cerebral palsy: Applying a WHO-ICF model. In: Proceedings of the 28th International Association of Logopedics and Phoniatrics, Athens, Greece, 2010 Aug 22-26.

[14] Hemphill L, Feldman HM, Camp L, Griffin TM, Miranda AE, Wolf DP. Developmental changes in narrative and non-narrative discourse in children with and without brain injury. J Commun Disord 1994;27(2):107-33.

[15] Nordberg A, Sandberg AD, Miniscalco C. Story retelling and language ability in school-aged children with cerebral palsy and speech impairment. Int J Lang Commun Disord 2015;50(6):801-13.

[16] Chengappa S, Bhat S, Iyer N. Mean length of utterance and syntactic complexity in the speech of the cerebral palsied. Lang India 2007;7(3):1-10.

[17] Gillam RB, Pearson NA. TNL: Test of narrative language. Austin, TX: PRO-ED Inc, 2004.

[18] Holck P, Nettelbladt U, Sandberg AD. Children with cerebral palsy, spina bifida and pragmatic language impairment: Differences and similarities in pragmatic ability. Res Dev Disabil 2009;30(5):942-51.

[19] Bottcher L. Children with spastic cerebral palsy, their cognitive functioning, and social participation: A review. Child Neuropsychol 2010;16(3):209-28.

[20] Leinonen E, Letts C, Smith BR. Children's pragmatic communication difficulties. London: Whurr publishers, 2000.

[21] Boudreau D. Narrative abilities: Advances in research and implications for clinical practice. Topics Lang Disord 2008;28(2):99-114.

[22] Hudson JA, Shapiro LR. From knowing to telling: The development of children's scripts, stories, and personal narratives. In: McCabe A, Peterson C, eds. Developing narrative structure. Hillsdale, NJ: Lawrence Erlbaum, 1991:89-136.

[23] Luciana M. Cognitive development in children born preterm: Implications for theories of brain plasticity following early injury. Dev Psychopathol 2003;15(4):1017-47.

[24] Straub K, Obrzut JE. Effects of cerebral palsy on neuropsychological function. J Dev Phys Disabil 2009;21(2):153-67.

[25] Norbury CF, Bishop DV. Inferential processing and story recall in children with communication problems: A comparison of specific language impairment, pragmatic language impairment and high-functioning autism. Int J Lang Commun Disord 2002;37(3):227-51.

[26] Brown R. A first language: The early stages. Cambridge, MA: Harvard University Press, 1973.

[27] Kramer CA, James SL, Saxman JH. A comparison of language samples elicited at home and in the clinic. J Speech Hear Disord 1979;44(3):321-30.

[28] Templin MC. Certain language skills in children; Their development and interrelationships. Westport, CT: Greenwood, 1957.

[29] Hess CW, Haug HT, Landry RG. The reliability of type-token ratios for the oral language of school age children. J Speech Hear Res 1989;32:536-40.

[30] Richards B. Type/token ratios: What do they really tell us? J Child Lang 1987;14(2):201-9.

[31] Blake J, Austin W, Cannon M, Lisus A, Vaughan A. The relationship between memory span and measures of imitative and spontaneous language complexity in preschool children. Int J Behav Dev 1994;17(1):91-107.

[32] Willis CS, Gathercole SE. Phonological short-term memory contributions to sentence processing in young children. Memory 2001;9(4-6):349-63.

In: Disability: International Aspects
Editors: Ariel Tenenbaum et al.
ISBN: 978-1-53617-886-9

Chapter 10

HOSTILITY AND VIOLENCE IMPEDING DEVELOPMENT OF CHILDREN WITH A DISABILITY: AN EXPERIENCE FROM BANGLADESH

Shaharior R Razu**, MA, Sheikh S Islam, MA and Dipak K Das, MA

Sociology Discipline, Khulna University,
Khulna and Department of English,
Northern University of Business and Technology,
Khulna, Bangladesh

ABSTRACT

Children with a disability can be victims of different forms of violence and hostility in society. This study attempts to describe how different types of hostility and violence experienced by children with a disability

---

* Corresponding Author: Shaharior R Razu, Assistant Professor, Sociology Discipline, Khulna University, Khulna, Bangladesh. E-mail: razusocku@gmail.com.

impede their physical and mental development. This chapter examines the nature, experiences, risk and impact of hostility and violence against children with disability. A qualitative approach was adopted for this study where data were collected through case studies, key informant interviews (KIIs) and focus group discussions (FGDs) from four schools for children with a disability in Khulna City of Bangladesh. A total of 24 respondents were selected from four randomly selected special-learning based schools of Khulna city including the children, their guardians and teachers. Findings indicated that children with a disability were victims of physical, mental, verbal and sexual violence both at home and in school. They, additionally, reported serious types of exclusion by their family members, relatives, neighbor and friends. As a result, they suffered from persistent biological, social and psychological problems which affected their normal life. The authors suggest that awareness, proper implementation of laws and special treatment are necessary for ensuring proper physical and mental development and protection of children with a disability in our society.

INTRODUCTION

Disability commonly refers to physical and/or mental impairment that restricts the normal functioning of people due to a wide range of health conditions (1, 2). Children with disability are those with such conditions which limits their life and puts them into a disadvantageous situation in society. These children can be subject to violence in different forms of abuse from the early days of their life (3). In spite of hardship, a child with disability has the potential to grow within his or her community and to affect the lives of the surrounding people (4). However, this fact is not always acknowledged as some people not only look down upon these special children, but also show hostility towards them. Additionally, there is increasing recognition of disparities experienced by these children, when compared with those without disabilities, including increased risks of violence (5). Therefore, unfriendliness and violence towards these children are occurring recurrently in our society. Discrimination in the family, community, workplace and other places is at the core of violations of the rights of children with disabilities (6). These children are victimized in two ways—as a disabled person and as a child. The impact of targeted violence and hostility is wide-ranging; in some instances, the experience can even result in the victim's death (3).

Children with disabilities are one of the most marginalized and excluded groups, experiencing widespread violations of their rights (7). They are usually perceived as disadvantaged groups by the society as well (8). The children with disabilities are feasibly being victims of child abuse, carelessness and ill-treatment. Different forms of targeted violence towards the disabled are observed in the forms of anti-social behavior, damage to property/theft, school bullying, incidents perpetrated by statutory agency staff and the most recent phenomenon of cyber bullying are widely prevalent these days (3). The children with disability can neither accept nor protest such behavior and often suffer from long term physical and psychological problems.

It is estimated that, about 10 percent of the world's children, which denotes some 200 million, have different types of impairment and 80 percent of them live in developing countries (9). Disability of a child is often monitored by its being marginalized in the society and it is found that only 2% of the children with disabilities have access to basic rights (10). They have to face various types of problem such as misbehavior, anti-social behavior or calling by name. They meet different forms of exclusion and are exaggerated to varying degrees of disability, where they live and the culture or class to which they belong (7). Like most of the developing countries, disabled children are at a higher risk of being victimized in comparison with non-disabled in Bangladesh. People in Bangladesh consider disability as a curse and a cause of humiliation to the family (11). There is an increasing risk of disabled children becoming unfortunate victims of violence due to their inability to defend themselves (10). The underestimation of the abilities of people with disabilities is a major obstacle to their inclusion and to the provision of equal opportunities (7).

These children are subject to targeted hostility and violence despite the different initiatives taken by both Government and Non-Government Organizations. Considering the importance of the issue, the present study attempted to explore the prevalent circumstance of the disabled children from a different perspective. For this, the following two research questions were taken into consideration— what is the nature of hostility and violence towards children with a disabilioty? And, which factors are influential to hostile attitude towards disabled children? The authors have tried to find the answers to the questions in the context of Khulna City of Bangladesh. Accordingly, this study attempts to showcase the violence against these children and make a clear understanding about the children with disabilities. We tried to gather information from the children themselves as well as their guardians and teachers to understand the nature of hostility and violence against them. Finally, we tried to find the impact of targeted violence and hostility on the physical and mental development of these children and suggest possible remedies for policy makers.

OUR STUDY

The present study is descriptive in nature and tries to identify how hostility and violence towards children with disabilities impact their physical and mental growth through a cross-sectional study. A qualitative approach was adopted for this study as it is generally more suitable for gaining more in-depth knowledge on the subject's individual experiences, beliefs, opinions, behaviors and feelings through empirical research. At first, four special-learning based schools were selected out of a total of eight special-learning schools located in Khulna City through simple random sampling for this study (see Table 1).

Table 1. List of the selected schools

Name of the schools	Location
Sarawar Autistic Children Welfare Organization (SACWO)	Basupara
SWID Intellectual Disabled School	Dalmil Mor
Hicare School and Hearing Centre	Boro Mirzapur
Hechac Hearing School	Babu Khan Road
Total Schools	4

After selecting those schools, a methodological triangulation of case studies, key informant interviews (KIIs), and focus group discussions (FGDs) were constructed for data collection. The unit of analysis for case studies was the children with disabilities of those four schools, yet considering the lack of their ability in interaction, their parents and teachers were selected as participants in KIIs. The authors conducted a total of six key informant interviews (KIIs) with three guardians and three teachers from the selected schools. Additionally, a couple of FGDs were conducted solely with two groups of children as we took eight participants in each session of those FGDs. As in qualitative studies credibility relies less on sample size rather on the richness of the gathered information and on the analytical abilities of the researcher, an optimum number of samples that was necessary for the study to reach a conclusion was selected. The participants were chosen through purposive and snowball sampling technique from the study area.

As key study instrument, separate interview schedules and check lists for all three modules of data collection were designed for this study. As case studies were the most intensive part of data collection in this study, individual interviews were carried out with the children in a number of sessions. Maintenance of equilibrium in participation from each of those four schools was prioritized by the authors as numbered each individual case (see Table 2).

Table 2. Participants of case studies

School name	Serial number of case study	Number of case study
Sarawar Autistic Children Welfare Organization (SACWO)	Case-1,2,3, 4, 5	5
SWID Intellectual Disabled School	Case- 6,7,8,9	4
Hicare School and Hearing Centre	Case- 10, 11, 12, 13	4
Hechac Hearing School	Case- 14, 15, 16, 17, 18	5
Total number of schools = 4		Total case study = 18

Table 3. Members of the focus group discussion

Category	Population category	Number of population from each schools
FGD	Sarawar Autistic Children Welfare Organization (SACWO)	2
	SWID Intellectual Disabled School	2
	Hicare School and Hearing Centre	2
	Hechac Hearing School	2
	Total number respondents in FGD	8

The FGDs provide essential information to understand not only what participants think, but also how and why they think that way. For this reason, a couple of FGDs, each composing eight members were conducted during the data collection phase. Principle of equality was maintained here as well as two disabled children from each of the four schools participated in those FGDs in two different sessions. The FGDs were conducted under the guidance of the chief investigator with the assistance of three trained moderators and two note takers. Table 3 shows the composition of the FGDs process for this study.

All data for this study were collected through the in-depth face-to-face interviews by dint of interview schedules, checklist, audio records and essential notes. The data collection continued over three months of duration starting in August, 2016 which continued till December, 2016. The authors analyzed and interpreted findings from case studies, FGDs and KIIs through the recorded documents for writing the research report.

Ethical considerations

As there are debates over ethical considerations about conducting studies with children (12), both written and verbal consent were acquired from each participant, their guardians, teachers and the concerned school authorities before data collection started for this study. The authors ensured strict standards of protecting privacy for personal information as they clarified the participants that the information collected will be used for the purpose of research only. All the participants were informed that the participation was voluntary and they have the liberty to terminate the interview at any point if they felt uncomfortable. Furthermore, the Academic Committee of the Sociology Discipline, Khulna University granted the ethical approval for this study.

Nature of hostility and violence

Children with disabilities often face a wide range of physical, mental, verbal and sexual violence. All the participants in the case studies, FGDs, and KIIs shared their opinion with the authors as they explained how surrounding people generally showed their attitude that were 'unfriendly' and 'unpleasant'. They believed that many people would find pleasure by teasing these children. Nahid Islam, a teenage boy, suffering from hearing disability, shared that some people find sarcastic pleasure from seeing his abnormal movement. He said:

> When I go outdoors, people of different ages and classes call me 'pagol' (mad) and talk about me with slackness and negligence. It seems to me that they are making fun of my abnormal behavior which makes me very sad.

In some cases, the children reported that their friends and classmates would laugh at them for no apparent reason. Their friends would share unwelcoming looks with them, and try to make fun of it. Their friends would never think that a child with disability is not responsible for their abnormality, and that he or she is not an object of laughter and ridicule. The mother of Santa Islam, a sixteen-year old partially mentally disabled girl, shared her experience in the following manner:

> ... we often feel ashamed of our disabled children in different situations, especially when some relatives visit our home. We are afraid

> that our child would do something wrong and they (the relatives) would start saying something embarrassing.

Many of the respondents in the case studies said that they generally face situations that are disturbing. They shared their experience of verbally aggressive approaches by others in roads and playgrounds. Like Santa added that some of her friends laugh at and tease her calling 'kufa' (ominous) and avoid her always. The authors also found that people often think that the disability of the children is a result of the sin of his or her parents. Sometimes they are deprived of human rights, and sometimes even they are exploited by their family members. In the absence of the proper support from the family members they feel insecure. Jahidul Islam, a visually disabled boy, for instance, faces discrimination and hostility within his family. His mother said:

> Even in my family, my husband sometimes misbehaves or hits him (Jahid) being out of temper. I don't think he is responsible for being abnormal? It is something we have no control over. I love my child very much for what he is. It is my fate and he is a blessing of Allah, I think.

The participants largely reported of all four forms of discrimination from their family as they did not the disabled member any different. These special children thought that they were of disgrace for the family, which made the disabled ashamed for the neglected behaviors from their relatives and neighbors. Sometimes even they reported that their playmates would scold them and torture them mentally without any reason. The stories of the participants revealed how unwelcoming attitude and hostile experiences ranged from their own family members to the outsides. Though shocking, this picture tells us the nature of violence thousands of disabled children experience every single day.

Experiences of the children with disability

The children are frequently treated negatively and considered a burden of the society. They are victims of physical, mental and sexual harassment. Even the disabled girls are the victims of teasing and inhuman physical domestic violence. Sometimes they try to protest, but the situations remain, because in any type of protest they do not usually get any type of support from anyone. One of the participants in FGDs, Meena, a ten year old partially disabled girl, shares how both familiar and unfamiliar people harass her in different situations because of her physical debility. She said:

> When someone laughs at and utters slung language because of my disability, I feel like crying. I even cannot say to my family. These incidents are really painful for me. Sometimes I feel like crying because of the negative attitudes from people. I try to do some work of my own, yet even my family members do not recognize my ability to do any work.

The researchers found that this girl was upset not for being physically challenged, but for the overall reception from the surrounding people. These types of gestures and comments dishearten her. Another participants, Shikta, stated:

> We are violated in an inhuman way and are excluded from every aspect of daily life. Nobody treats us normally, be it family or outsiders. I have multiple first-hand experiences of such behavior and trust me it is painful."

From their first hand experiences, the children realize that society does not want them. They are a burden for the society. Very few people encourage the abilities of these children. They remain unnoticed and ignored in all spheres of life. The same way, many special children are treated in an adverse way which destroys their positive attitude towards life. Some even do not find any meaning in their lives, and do not understand why they are surviving. They suffer from extreme pessimism, which destroys all the productivity they possess. Thus the society is deprived of the service they would render for it.

Risk factors

The authors recorded some stories of intimidating attitudes from both the known and unknown people experienced by the children. These negative approaches involved greater risks for a normal life of the disabled. A study suggested that disability increases potential threats for children in a number of ways (13). Extreme physical and mental pressure is a critical menace for the future of this vulnerable group. As they have less opportunity for proper education and jobs, they cannot participate in any social activities and are deprived of basic human needs and rights. The authors noted that the children had a lack of access to psychological mental health support, which was also found in some other studies (14, 15). The children often seemed to be in the midst of hesitation and lack of confidence throughout the study. One of the teachers at SWID Intellectual Disabled School who participated in KIIs, Zihad Ahmed, said:

> … they are often treated unfairly as they always remain in vulnerable to ill experiences. There is a prodigious chance of being physically detached from the society for them. I have dealt a number of cases where this detachment makes them extremely pessimistic. Such experiences may deter the normal growth for them.

The thing is that in spite of having potentials they lose hope, because of the attitudes of the surrounding people. Sometimes their near and dear ones encourage them and nourish them to some extent, yet the approaches of other people discourage them. Ms Rawshan Ara, one of the teachers who participated in the key informant interviews (KIIs) discussed another type of prevalent risk of such children. She thinks that the continuous negative approach towards a physically challenged child will push him or her to a state of susceptibility and destruction, and in addition, will increase their disability. To quote her words:

> Continuous violence against disabled children put a negative impact on them. Most of the time, they lose their self-confidence due to such an attitude. These make them more vulnerable and accelerate their disability, delay their cognitive development, psychological improvement and create various types of problems.

Her fear is not a counterfeit. Rather, it really happens to them. They are helpless to get rid of this problem, and they embrace a risky future, both for themselves and the society. Tania Ahmed, another participant, added some other risky situations that these children would face. In her opinion, the prevalent surliness towards them may result in a hindrance in their socialization. As they fail to adopt themselves with other children and people there create an excessive gap between the children and the rest of the people of the society.

Impact of hostility and violence

There are both long-term and short-term impacts of negative attitudes and treatment on the children. The children are treated worthlessly in the society and perceived as they are not eligible for any work. The hostility and violence that they undergo hamper both their psychological and physical growth. When someone laughs at them without any logical reason, they feel humiliated, but cannot realize the reason of the laughter. Then they start thinking that they are a subject of fun and ridicule. They even start avoiding public spaces, where they perceive potential threats of bullying and maltreatment (16). Such a picture represents how enormous mental stress they have to bear every day. Anjuman Ara, a teacher of Hicare School and Hearing Centre, shared her experience:

> When treated adversely, the mental growth of the children is deterred significantly. We see major psychological problems such as lack of

confidence, depression, anxiety and even deviant behavior amongst the disabled children because of long term ill-treatment

Research suggests that hostility and unfriendliness may leave a long lasting influence on the children (17). It destroys their future and ruins their present. Such experience also may make a child less sociable and leave permanent personality disorder. Due to unfriendly attitudes the children start feeling isolated. The idea of becoming self-dependent remains unattainable for them.

Such attitudes, in fact, destroy their potentials on the one hand, and they cannot lead a happy life in line with the normal children, on the other. Another impact of violence and hostility towards these children is that as in many cases they have potentials, yet society cannot get the fruitfulness of that. In this respect, Halima Akter, a teacher of Sarawar Autistic Children Welfare Organization (SACWO) said, sometimes the disabled children have much potentiality than that of the normal children, but the society do not accept them warmly and their development process faces obstacles and the potentiality cannot flourish. She added:

> The disabled children are in the most vulnerable situation and are at risk. As the society does not accept them, the ultimate sufferer will be the society because, perhaps, it will lose a good teacher or scientist or any type of the best professional for their ignorance.

The picture shows that these children can hardly avoid the adverse impacts on them. The impact of such treatment may result in serious physical and mental issues. Due to several supercilious attitudes and the lack of proper support and treatment many physically disabled children—both physical and mental disability—deteriorate in an alarming speed. Additionally, they cannot help themselves in their development, and they cannot contribute for the betterment of the society at large. Throughout their life span they lead a very pathetic life. The authors identified some of the major impacts of such experience on disabled children as followed:

- Long-term mental effects (e.g., depression, anxiety, frustration, lack of confidence etc.)
- Loss of physical health
- Limiting the life chances
- Avoiding tendencies (less sociability and gregariousness)
- Aggressive and deviant behavior etc.

DISCUSSION

This paper investigates the nature, risk, prevalence and impact of targeted hostility and violence towards children with disabilities in Bangladesh. As the paper addresses all aspects related to hostility and violence towards these children, findings represent what kind of violence are experienced by the children with disabilities, who are responsible for this, which place are risky for them, how vulnerable they are and how much the children are squeezed by the hostility and violence. Their vulnerable condition is generated from a number of factors—the identification of which gets next priority of the research objective. Besides, the role of family, educational, religious and political institutions is questioned for improving this marginalized section of the society.

The study identifies that all the participants stated that children with disabilities have a very limited or no access to basic child rights. They face substantial difficulties in enjoying their essential rights such as vital foods, proper clothing, education, health facilities and so on. They are the marginalized groups who are not able to get health related information properly (18). Except special schools for these children, general schools are not designed to support the children with disabilities and the teachers are not adequately trained. In this situation, children with disabilities are likely to face serious challenges to get education (19). Additionally, the children with disabilities often face maltreatments, because of their disability (18). They are the victim of misbehavior of their near ones who are supposed to take care of them.

It is widely observed that the children suffer from various types of unfriendly attitudes from not only strangers, but also the people surrounding them. They are victimized, because many perpetrators seek individuals who are unable to understand and communicate criminal actions. Beaten by family members or peer groups, pushed by friends in schools or by anonymous on street/public transport is some of the common physical violence happening to them. Sometimes, family members harass them, but also unknown people are involved in the hostility and violence towards them. Therefore, functioning of parents is related highly to the emotional functioning of children. Sexual abuse and harassment are more common against children with disabilities. It is estimated that 1.8 million children are being sexually exploited, while three-fourth of them are girls (20-22).

In our society, disabled children are at a greater risk, because of two specific minority traits. First, they are children and second, they are disabled. So, they are actually double victims. It is evident that hostility and violence are serious problems for children with disabilities, who are at a greater risk than the normal children (23, 24). The prevalence rate of exposure to violence for children with disabilities was 3.6% in comparison to children without disabilities who has a prevalence rate of 2.1% indicating the noticeable and significant difference in exposure to acts of violence. Disabled children are not safe outside home, such as in school, at playground, on street or in public transport.

The impact of hostility and violence towards disabled children may result in tremendous confusion and frustration for them (25) and for this they might feel angry, sad, lonely, frustrated, or hopeless as a result of focusing on their difficulties (26). They also feel agitated, helpless, fear to disclosure, despondency and this may make a sense of abhorrence of life which results committing suicide. Problems associated with exposure to violence for anyone include injury, death, depression, anxiety, alcohol/drug use, eating disorders, sleep-disorders, stress-related symptoms, gastrointestinal problems, migraines, suicide ideation/attempts, and post-traumatic stress disorder (27). Disabled children, who face serious types of hostility and violence, are not interested to communicate with others or go outside home. They try to avoid the place where they face problems as well as they try to avoid the wrongdoer. The hostility and violence not only affect their feeling and interest, but also can be cause of their severe physical and mental injury. Specifically, these consequences may include wound to the nervous system, cracks, and damage to the inner organs of body.

CONCLUSION

Disabled children are being victimized by targeted violence, which deters their mental and physical growth significantly. In this study, the authors identified how they are victimized by different forms of violence from their family, relatives, neighbor, peer groups, and also outsiders. Such experience leaves a permanent impact on their physical, mental and social life. Some of these major impacts include fear, isolation, tendency to suicide, feeling of inferiority, personality disorder etc. Sometimes targeted violence towards may lead the disabled to aggressive and deviant behavior. The scenario should be changed through formulating effective child rights laws and implementing them. Besides, a wide circulation of information is necessary for building-up awareness among the people. Arrangement for special education, training and supervision can help improve the situation as it will help the disabled for becoming self-dependant. Most importantly, the family and surrounding institutions have a greater role to play by making a harmonious environment and acceptance for these special children.

REFERENCES

[1] Mitchell, G. Children with disabilities using child and family welfare services. OzChild 2013. URL: https://www.ozchild.org.au/wp-content/uploads/2015/03/OzChild_DisabilityResearchReport_2014.pdf.

[2] WHO. Disability: Report by the secretariat to the 132 session of the executive board. Geneva: World Health Organisation, 2012. URL: 07apps.who.int/gb/ebwha/pdf_files/WHA66/A66_12-en.pdf.
[3] Sin CH, Hedges A, Cook C, Mguni N, Comber N. Disabled people's experiences of targeted violence and hostility. Manchester: Equality Human Rights Commission, 2009.
[4] Tran KV. Exploring the experience of children with disabilities at school settings in Vietnam context. SpringerPlus 2013;3(103):1-10.
[5] Jones L, Bellis MA, Wood S, Hughes K, McCoy E, Eckley L. Prevalence and risk of violence against children with disabilities: a systematic review and meta-analysis of observational studies. Lancet 2012;380(9845):899–907.
[6] UNICEF. Situation analysis on children with disabilities in Bangladesh 2014. Dhaka: UNICEF Bangladesh, 2014.
[7] UNICEF. Children and young people with disabilities: Fact Sheet 2013. New York: UNICEF, 2013.
[8] Block ME. What is appropriate physical education for students with profound disabilities? Adapt Phys Act Q 1992;9:197-213.
[9] UNICEF. Promoting the rights of children with disabilities. Florence: Innocenti Research Center, 2007.
[10] Titumir RAM, Hossain J. Disability in Bangladesh: Prevalence, knowledge, attitude and practices. Unnayan Onneshan 2005;1:1-98.
[11] Patton MQ. Qualitative evaluation and research methods, Third edition. Thousand Oaks, CA: Sage, 2002.
[12] Lindsay G. Researching children's perspectives: Ethical issues. Researching children's perspectives. Buckingham: Open University Press, 2000.
[13] Petersilia J. Invisible victims: violence against persons with developmental disabilities. Hum Rights 2000;27:1:9.
[14] Peckham NG, Corbett A, Howlett S., McKee A, Pattison S. The delivery of a survivor. Group for learning disabled women with significant learning disabilities who have been sexually abused. Br J Learn Disabil 2007;35,4:236–44.
[15] Sequeira H. Implications for practice: research into the effects of sexual abuse on adults with intellectual disabilities. J Adult Prot 2006;8,4:25-34.
[16] Mencap. Bullying wrecks lives: The experiences of children and young people with a learning disability. London: Mencap, 2007.
[17] Hunter C, Hodge N, Nixon J, Parr S, Willis B. Disabled people's experiences of anti-social behaviour and harassment in social housing: A critical review. London: Disability Rights Commission, 2007.
[18] Uromi SM, Mazagwa MI. Challenges facing people with disabilities and possible solutions in Tanzania. J Educ Policy Entre Res 2014;1(2):158-65.
[19] Mpofu E, Kasayira JM, Mhaka MM, Chireshe R, Maunganidze L. Inclusive Zimbabwe. In: Engelbert P, Green L, eds. Responding to the challenges of inclusive education in Southern Africa. Pretoria, SA: Van Schaik, 2007.

[20] Finkelhor D. Child sexual abuse. In: Rosenberg M, Fenley MA, eds. Violence in America: A public health approach. New York: Oxford University Press, 1991.

[21] Finkelhor D, Williams LM. Burns N. Nursery crimes: Sexual abuse in day care. Newbury Park, CA: Sage, 1988.

[22] Finkelhor D. A sourcebook on child sexual abuse. Newbury Park, CA: Sage, 1986.

[23] Brown H, Stein J, Turk V. The sexual abuse of adults with learning disabilities: Report of a second two-year incidence survey. Ment Handicap Res 1995;8(1):3-24.

[24] Goldson E. Invited commentary: Children with disabilities and child maltreatment. Child Abuse Negl 1998;22:663-7.

[25] Pizzi J. Challenges of children with physical disabilities. Rivier Acad J 2008;4(1): 1-9.

[26] Neeraja P, Anuradha K. Adjustment problems faced by children with learning disabilities impact of special education. Indian J Sci Res 2014;5(1):77-81.

[27] American Psychological Association. Violence and the family: Report of the American Psychological Association Presidential Task Force on Violence and the Family. Washington DC: APA, 1996.

In: Disability: International Aspects
Editors: Ariel Tenenbaum et al.
ISBN: 978-1-53617-886-9

Chapter 11

NEEDS FOR ASSISTIVE DEVICES AND ENVIRONMENTAL MODIFICATION IN THAI PERSONS WITH DISABILITIES: ARE THERE DIFFERENCES BETWEEN YOUNGER AND OLDER AGE GROUPS?

Buakarn Kayaphard[1], MD
and Jittima Saengsuwan[2]*, MD, PhD
[1]Rehabilitation Medicine Unit, Khon Kaen hospital,
Khon kaen, Thailand
[2]Department of Rehabilitation Medicine, Faculty of Medicine,
Khon Kaen University, Khon Kaen, Thailand

ABSTRACT

Worldwide, there are increasing numbers of people with a disability. There is limited study on persons with disabilities (PWD) perspective of

---

* Corresponding Author: Jittima Saengsuwan, MD, PhD, Department of Rehabilitation Medicine, Faculty of Medicine, Khon Kaen University, Khon Kaen, 40002, Thailand. E-mail: sjittima@kku.ac.th.

their own needs and no study has previously compared the differing needs between younger and older PWD. Objective: This chapter has twofold aims: To determine the PWD perspective on the need for assistive devices and environmental intervention; and to determine the difference between younger and older PWD in aspect of their needs. Methods: A cross-sectional face-to-face interview study with 409 PWDs in two main districts in Khon Kaen Province, North-Eastern Thailand. Data were collected from March 2015-March 2016. Results: The mean age of PWD was 59.3 ± 17.2 years (range 18-102 years). Highest needs reported were mobility aids (13.9%), hearing aids (9.3%), visual aids and prosthesis (8.8% each). The older age group reported double the needs for most assistive devices and for carers over the younger group: e.g., Need for mobility aids (17.7% vs 9.5%) and hearing aids (12.7% vs 5.3%) respectively. A quarter (24.7%) of PWD reported that they need home modifications. Conclusion: Results suggest limited access to health care support services. The high perceived need for assistive devices and environmental interventions indicates that there is an urgent need for enhancing national policy to improve health care support services for PWD.

INTRODUCTION

Worldwide, it is estimated that there are approximately 650 million people with a disability. Of these, 110 million people have difficulty in daily living (1). According to a 2012 Thai survey, it was estimated there were 1.5 million people living with disability, 2.2% of the whole country. 1.4 million persons noted limitation in social participation and approximately 0.3 million people noted difficulty in taking care of selves (2). There were more females than males and the largest group with disability was the over 70 year age group. The most common disability was physical disability, which accounted for nearly half of the whole disability population in both younger and older age groups (2). As older age was associated with an increasing chance of being disabled, the current and future situation of PWD in Thailand is worrisome as the number of elderly is growing rapidly. Currently, 16% of the total Thai population are elderly. This number is estimated to increase to over 30% of the total population by 2035 (3).

The United Nations' Convention on the Rights of Person with Disabilities (CRPD) aimed to promote, protect and ensure the full and equal enjoyment of all human rights and fundamental freedoms by all persons with disabilities, and to promote respect for their inherent dignity. In Chapter 4 of CRPD the topic related to assistive devices states that States' parties should provide accessible information to persons with disabilities about mobility aids, devices and assistive technologies, including new technologies, as well as other forms of assistance, support services and facilities (4). In relation to the CRPD, in Thailand there is the Empowerment of Persons with Disabilities Act, B.E. 2550 (2007) which aimed to support and to improve quality of life in PWD as well as to ensure their human rights and fundamental freedoms (5). Part of section 20 in this act states that PWD have the rights to access and utilize public facilities including welfare services and other supports from the government such as medical rehabilitation, assistive devices as well as modification of housing environment. Further, this Act advises the health care sectors to prepare themselves for the rise in PWD who need the assistive devices or access to other health care services to ensure accessibility.

Physical disability exerts a negative impact on education, work and community life. It is found that assistive technology such as wheelchair can have a positive socioeconomic effect on the lives of people with disability by increasing their educational accessibility, work participation and health maintenance (6, 7). According to previous study regarding gait aid uses in elderly, it was found that the usage rate was high and high degrees of effectiveness was found. Gait aids increased safety and decreased effort for various activities (8). Having a chance to get the assistive device may lessen dependency and improving quality of life in older PWD. To date, there are very limited resources studying the accessibility or the need of person with disability (PWD). Borg et al. (9) stated that needs of assistive device varies greatly between countries and regions within countries. The authors also emphasized that needs assessment is a prerequisite to plan services (9). Since the profiles and needs of older people with disability may differ from younger age group, it is crucial to explore the need of older PWD to plan the health service and support.

There has been limited study on PWD perspective of needs and no Thai study has previously compared the difference in needs between younger and older people with physical disability. Therefore, the aims of this study were twofold: to investigate Thai PWD perspective on the need for assistive devices and environmental intervention; and to determine the difference between younger and older PWD in aspect of their needs.

OUR STUDY

This cross-sectional community-based questionnaire survey study was approved by the Ethics Review Committee of Khon Kaen Hospital, Thailand (KE60082). The study was carried out between March 2015-March 2016, in two major districts (Muang and Banpai Districts) with a combined population of 242,322, from Khon Kaen Province, North Eastern Thailand (total provincial population of 1,801,753) (10).

Participants

This study was a part of the main disability survey which includes total of 1007 persons with various forms of disability (mental, visual impairment, deaf, intellectual disability and physical disability) whose names are registered in the PWD district data. Four hundred and nine patients met our inclusion criteria. The inclusion criteria were, participants must be 1) registered with a physical disablility, 2) be older than 18 years and 3) not have a cognitive or communication problem.

Demographic data (gender, age, family members, monthly income), disability profiles (type of disability, complications), needs for assistive devices, need for modification of home/work place, education, work, social participation and the care they have received were also recorded.

Data collection

Fifteen home health care personnel, trained for looking after people with disability in community had 6 hours additional interviewer training including theory and practice by nurses, a physical therapist and public health staff. The home health care personnel visited people with registered disability and had 30-60-minute face-to-face interviews with the questionnaire.

Data analysis

Data were analysed using SPSS (V 20.0, IBM Corp., Armonk, NY). Continuous variables were presented as mean ± standard deviation (SD) if the data were normally distributed and median (interquartile range) if the data were not normally distributed. Categorical variables were presented as frequencies and percentages. Normality of continuous data was tested by Shapiro-Wilk test. To compare between younger (less than or equal to 60 years) and older age group (more than 60 years), t-test was used if the data were normally distributed and Kruskal-Wallis test was used if the data were not normally distibuted. For comparison of the proportion between 2 groups, chi-square test was used and if there were data with less than 5 in a cell, Fisher's exact test was used. The cutoff point of 60 years old is offical retirement age and considered old age in Thailand. The significance level was set at 0.05.

Findings

Four hundred and nine persons with disabilities (PWD) were interviewed for the study with an almost even male/female split (males 52.3%). The mean age was 59.3 years (range 18-102 years). A higher proportion of female PWDs (56.8%) was found in the older age group; males prediminated in younger age group (60.8%).

Table 1. Participant demographics (n = 409)

Variables	Total (n = 409)	18-60 years (n = 189)	>60 years (n = 220)	P-value
Female	199 (48.7%)	74 (39.2%)	125 (56.8%)	<0.001
Age, mean (SD)	59.3 (17.2)	44.0 (11.3)	72.5 (7.9)	NA
range	19-102	19-60	61-102	
Education:				
No education	52 (12.7%)	29 (15.3%)	23(7.5%)	<0.001
Primary school	298 (72.9%)	118 (62.4%)	180 (81.9%)	
Secondary school	44 (10.8%)	30 (20.6%)	14 (6.4%)	
Higher education	13 (3.2%)	11 (5.8%)	2 (1%)	
Missing	2 (0.004%)	1(0.5%)	1 (0.5%)	
Marital status:				
Married	191 (46.7%)	74 (39.2%)	117 (53.2%)	<0.001
Single	108 (26.4%)	97 (51.3%)	11 (5%)	
Widowed	93 (22.7%)	8 (4.2%)	85 (38.6%)	
Divorced	12 (2.9%)	9 (4.8%)	3 (1.4%)	
Missing	5 (1.2%)	1 (0.5%)	4 (1.8%)	
Pre-disability occupation				
Study	4 (1%)	4 (2.2%)	0 (0%)	<0.001
Employed	323 (79.0%)	133 (70.4%)	190 (86.4%)	
Unemployed	76 (18.6%)	50 (26.4%)	26 (11.8%)	
Missing	6 (1.5%)	2 (1.1%)	4 (1.8%)	
Median pre-disability income (IQR) (Baht)	2000 (3625)	3000 (4200)	2000 (1600)	0.25
Post-disability occupation				
Employed	149 (36.4%)	92 (48.7%)	85 (38.6%)	<0.001
Unemployed	244 (59.7%)	88 (46.6%)	128 (58.1%)	
Missing	16 (3.9%)	9 (4.8%)	7 (3.2%)	
Median postdisability income (IQR) (Baht)	2215 (950)	800 (2200)	1500 (200)	<0.001
Underlying diseases	145 (35.5%)	37 (19.6%)	108 (49.1%)	<0.001
Complications:	58 (14.2%)	15 (7.9%)	43 (19.5%)	<0.001
Joint stiffness	41 (10.0%)	8 (4.2%)	33 (15%)	0.63
Pressure ulcers	4 (0.01%)	2 (1.1%)	2 (0.9%)	0.27
Family members, Mean (SD)	4.0 (1.9)	4.0 (1.9)	4.0 (2.0)	0.93
Caregiver				
No caregiver	12 (2.4%)	8 (4.2%)	4 (1.8%)	0.33
Relatives	379 (92.7%)	172 (42.1%)	207 (94.1%)	
missing	18 (4.4%)	9 (4.8%)	9 (4.1%)	
Social participation	256 (62.6%)	112 (59.3%)	144 (65.5%)	0.16
Religion participation	258 (63.1%)	120 (63.5%)	138 (62.7%)	0.56

Most had less than secondary schooling (95.6%) and were unemployed (59.7%). Nearly half were married (46.7%). However, in younger PWD they were more likely to be single (51.3%). A higher percentage of older PWDs were married (53.2%) or widowed (38.6%). Older PWD had higher post disability income (median 1500 bht ($450)) compared to younger age group (median 800 bht($240)) because the government supports more money for people who are more than 60 years. Older PWD had concurrent underlying disease (49.1 vs 19.6%) and reported complications (19.5% vs 7.9%) compared to younger PWD. However, there was no significant difference in the proportion of PWD with joint stiffness and pressure ulcers between both groups. Most had their relatives as their caregivers. There was no difference between younger and older PWD in the proportion of PWD who participated in social and religious events (see Table 1).

Needs reported and difference between younger and older PWD in aspect of needs in assistive devices

Mobility aids (13.9%), hearing aids (9.3%), prostheses (8.8%) and visual aids (8.8%) ranked highest as perceived assistive device needs. Perceived need for hearing aids and mobility aids were significantly higher in older age group (see Table 2).

Table 2. Reported needs for assistive devices

Variables	Total (n = 409)	18-60 years (n = 189)	>60 years (n = 220)	P-value
Mobility aids	57 (13.9%)	18 (9.5%)	39 (17.7%)	0.054
Hearing aids	38 (9.3%)	10 (5.3%)	28 (12.7%)	0.03
Prosthesis	36 (8.8%)	13 (6.9%)	23 (10.5%)	0.21
Visual aids	36 (8.8%)	13 (6.9%)	23 (10.5%)	0.21
Carers	24 (5.9%)	6 (3.2%)	18 (8.2%)	0.09
Diapers or urinary catheter	16 (3.9%)	5 (2.6%)	11 (5%)	0.15
Others	7 (1.7%)	1 (0.5%)	6 (2.7%)	0.10
Braces or shoes	5 (1.2%)	3 (1.6%)	2 (0.9%)	0.16

Table 3. Reported needs for environmental modification

Variables	Total	18-60 years (n = 189)	>60 years (n = 220)	
Home				
Home modification	101 (24.7%)	42 (22.2%)	59 (26.8%)	0.49
Toilet modification	71 (17.4%)	30 (15.9%)	41 (18.6%)	0.67
Ramp	33 (8.1%)	16 (8.5%)	17 (7.7%)	0.87
Bedroom modification	34 (8.3%)	17 (9.0%)	17 (7.7%)	0.30
Work				
Disability hindered work	80 (19.6%)	48 (25.4%)	32 (14.6%)	<0.001
Office modification	28 (6.9%)	20 (10.6%)	8 (3.7%)	0.006
Toilet modification	30 (7.4%)	21 (11.1%)	11 (5.0%)	0.033
Work modification	48 (11.8%)	30 (15.9%)	18 (8.2%)	0.026
Carer	28 (6.9%)	19 (10.1%)	9 (4.1%)	0.039
New occupational training	27 (6.6%)	20 (10.6%)	7 (3.2%)	0.003
Social				
Socialize	155 (38%)	73 (38.6%)	82 (37.4%)	0.08
Place PWD would like to go most:	(n = 336)	(n = 155)	(n = 181)	
Temple	261 (77.7%)	107 (69.0%)	154 (85.1%)	<0.001
Market	36 (10.7%)	30 (19.4%)	6 (3.3%)	0.31
Hospital	35 (10.4%)	19 (12.3%)	16 (8.5%)	<0.001
Social space modification	56 (13.7%)	29 (15.3%)	27 (12.3%)	0.38
Toilet modification	73 (17.9%)	34 (18.0%)	39 (17.8%)	0.96
Carer	62 (15.2%)	27 (14.3%)	35 (16.0%)	0.80
Help to enable out	41 (10%)	21 (11.1%)	20 (9.1%)	0.51

Table 4. Reported reasons for not having home modifications

Variables	Total (n = 101)	18-60 years (n = 42)	>60 years (n = 59)	p-value
Lack of money	81 (80.2%)	33 (78.6%)	48 (81.4%)	0.80
Lack of knowledge	51 (50.5%)	17 (40.4%)	34 (57.6%)	0.09
Don't have right to do/ not own house	6 (5.9%)	5 (11.9%)	1 (1.7%)	0.03

A quarter of PWD reported the need for home modification (24.7%), especially toilet modifications (17.4%). No significant difference was found between the two age groups in expressed need for home modifications. Lack of knowledge (80.2%) and lack of money (50.5%) were considered the main obstacles for environmental intervention. Not owning their own house was considered a limitation for modifying the environment by 12% of younger PWDs. Younger PWD found disabilty to limit their employment chances. The need to modify the work place was significantly higher in the younger age group compared to older age group for all aspects of work (need to modify offices, toilets, work practices, and need to alter carreers, and for new occupational training). Nearly 40% of PWD reported needing help to enhance socialization. The highest rated modification to enhance socialization was toilet modification (17.9%). Most PWD (77.7%) rated temple as the place they would like to go, followed by market and hospital.

DISCUSSION

We found that mobility aids, hearing aids, prosthetics devices and visual aids were most commonly quoted assistive devices needed. The older PWD requirements of assistive devices were two fold higher than in younger PWD. The higher needs for assistive devices in elderly PWD supported the previous findings that older people have limited accessibility to health care support systems, for example, lack of ability to independently access to the health care system (7).

In Thailand, the accessibility for PWD to get the assistive devices is limited. Approximately 14.0-15.0% of PWD did not have a chance to access to the assistive devices provided by the health care system (2, 7). Kulpeng et al. (7) estimated the economic loss of not having chance to get to the assistive device cost the lost of 2,497 million baht per year as the use of assistive device can enable PWD to be independent, to make a living to support themselves and their family (7).

Assistive device together with environmental intervention can reduce in-home personnel cost as well as institutional care cost (11). Although environmental modification intervention did not change dependency, evidence shows that environmental modification provides a long lasting effect of reduction of person's level of difficulty in both activities of daily living and instrumental activities of daily living especially bathing and toileting in older adults with chronic conditions (12, 13). Moreover, the positive effect was also applied to the caregiver as it enhance caregiver self-efficacy and reduces upset in some area of caregiving in patient with dementia (14).

Regarding the need for environmental modification, there was no significant difference for the requirement of home and social place modifications in younger and older age groups. The most commonly required modification was toilet for both home and social space. A quarter of patients reported the need for home modification. The most common causes of not modifying home were lack of money and lack of knowledge, respectively.

There was significantly higher requirement for work place modification for younger PWD. A quarter of younger PWD perceived that disability hindered their work. The younger PWD had significantly higher needs for office modifications, toilet modification at work place, work modification, carer and new occupation training compared to older PWD. Nearly 40% of PWD reported need for socialization and the highest rated need was for going to the temple (77.7%), reflecting the influence of culture.

The high need for assistive devices and environmental interventions found in this study especially in older PWD clearly indicates that there is an urgent need to provide a national policy to promote adequate accessibility of care in PWD. Additionally, long term plan to provide an appropriate system to support PWD at the time of high demand for these should be considered for the future.

In summary, there are still problems for Thai PWD with access to health care support services and lack of home modifications although the demand for these are high. The issues of accessibility and chance of home modifications should to be discussed and included in future government policy development plans.

Limitations

This study had several limitations. Firstly, the results from this study may not be generalizable because needs of assistive device varies between countries and regions within countries (9). Secondly, this study was based on patient's perspective of needs thus the results may be underestimated when compared to what healthcare professionals evaluated.

CONCLUSION

Being old doubled the neeed for assistive devices compared to younger PWD. The most commonly requested assistive devices were mobility aids, hearing aids, prosthetics and visual aids. The highest rated needs for home and social space modification were for toilets. The highest perceived needs, for assistive devices and environmental interventions, indicates that there is an urgent need to provide a national policy to improve health care support systems for PWD.

ACKNOWLEDGMENTS

We would like to thank all the people with disabilities and health care personnel who took the time to participate in this research. We would like to acknowledge Associate Professor John F Smith for English editing of the manuscript via the Publication Clinic KKU, Thailand. This study was supported by Thai Health Promotion Foundation (Ref. 59-00-104). The authors declare no conflict of interest.

REFERENCES

[1] World Health Organization. World report on disability. Geneva: World Health Organization, 2011.

[2] National Statistical Office. The 2012 disability survey. URL: http://service.nso.go.th/nso/nsopublish/themes/files/disabled55.pdf.

[3] Knodel J, Teerawichitchainan B, Prachuabmoh V, Pothisiri W. The situation of Thailand's older population. An updated based on the 2014 survey of older persons in Thailand. Ann Arbor, MI: Population Studies Center, Institue for Social Research, University of Michigan, 2015.

[4] United Nations. Convention on the Rights of Person with Disabilities. Resolution 61/106. New York: United Nations, 2007.

[5] National Office for Empowerment of Persons with Disability. Persons with disabilities empowerment act B.E. 2550. Bangkok: NEP, 2007.

[6] Borg J, Larsson S, Ostergren PO, Rahman A, Bari N, Khan A. Assistive technology use and human rights enjoyment: a cross-sectional study in Bangladesh. BMC Int Health Human Rights 2012;12:18.

[7] Kulpeng W, Kingkaew P, Kaewsawang S, Tantivess S, Teerawattananon Y. Outcomes and factors influencing access to assistive device for mobility disabled people. J Health Systems Res 2015;9:344-57.

[8] Sonn U, Grimby G. Assistive devices in an elderly population studied at 70 and 76 years of age. Disabil Rehabil 1994;16:85-92.

[9] Borg J, Lindstrom A, Larsson S. Assistive technology in developing countries: national and international responsibilities to implement the Convention on the Rights of Persons with Disabilities. Lancet 2009;374:1863-5.

[10] Official Statistics Registration Systems. Population and housing statistics. URL: http://stat.dopa.go.th/stat/statnew/upstat_age.php.

[11] Mann W, Ottenbacher K, Fraas L, Tomita M, Granger C. Effectiveness of assistive technology and environmental interventions in maintaining independence and reducing home care costs for frail elderly. A randomized controlled trial. Arch Fam Med 1999;8:210-7.

[12] Gitlin LN, Winter L, Dennis MP, Corcoran M, Schinfeld S, Hauck WW. A randomized trial of a multicomponent home intervention to reduce functional difficulties in older adults. J Am Geriatrics Soc 2006;54:809-16.

[13] Petersson I, Lilja M, Hammel J, Kottorp A. Impact of home modification services on ability in everyday life for people ageing with disabilities. J Rehabil Med 2008;40:253-60.

[14] Gitlin LN, Corcoran M, Winter L, Boyce A, Hauck WW. A randomized, controlled trial of a home environmental intervention: Effect on efficacy and upset in caregivers and on daily function of persons with dementia. Gerontologist 2001;41:4-14.

In: Disability: International Aspects
Editors: Ariel Tenenbaum et al.
ISBN: 978-1-53617-886-9

Chapter 12

OROFACIAL INJURIES AMONGST COMMERCIAL MOTORCYCLISTS, DRIVERS, AND BUS CONDUCTORS IN THREE RURAL COMMUNITIES, SOUTH-WESTERN NIGERIA

Kehinde K Kanmodi[1-4,*], BDS, AISQEM,
Olatunji A Lawal[1,5], BDS,
Zainab O Akintola[1,6], BDS
and Olushola Ibiyemi[1,2,7], BDS, MPH, PhD, FMCDS

[1]Department of Periodontology and Community Dentistry, University of Ibadan, Ibadan, Nigeria
[2]Cephas Health Research Initiative Inc, Ibadan, Nigeria
[3]Department of Dental and Maxillofacial Surgery, Usmanu Danfodiyo University Teaching Hospital, Sokoto, Nigeria
[4]Community Health Officers Training Programme, Usmanu Danfodiyo University Teaching Hospital, Sokoto, Nigeria
[5]Dental Centre, University College Hospital, Ibadan, Nigeria

[*] Correspondence: Kehinde Kanmodi, BDS, Cephas Health Research Initiative Inc, Sokoto, Nigeria. Email: kanmodikehinde@yahoo.com.

[6]Dental Department, Oyo State Hospital Management Board, Ibadan, Nigeria
[7]Department of Periodontology and Community Dentistry, University College Hospital, Ibadan, Nigeria

ABSTRACT

In this chapter we want to determine the prevalence, pattern, and psychosocial impact of orofacial injuries among commercial motorcyclists, drivers, and bus conductors in rural Eruwa, Lanlate, and Igboora communities, Nigeria. Methods: A cross-sectional study was undertaken among 100 randomly selected study participants who resided in Eruwa, Lanlate and Igboora communities, Nigeria. A pre-tested semi-structured questionnaire was used to interview the consenting participants. Data was analysed using the SPSS version 16 software. Results: All the respondents were males and their mean (±SD) age was 32.22 (±8.79) years. The majority (77%) of them were married, 55% had secondary school education, and 62% were motorcyclists. Only 42% of the respondents had never consumed alcohol, while 90% had never consumed tobacco. When on highway, only 26 (72.2%) of the drivers use seat belt always, none of the bus conductors had ever used seat belt, and only 3 (4.8%) of the motorcyclists wear helmet always. Only eight (8%) and five (5%) study respondents had histories of automobile crash-related oral and facial injuries respectively. Overall, a higher proportion of those with oral injuries had associated psychosocial problems, unlike those with facial injuries. Conclusion: The prevalence of oral and facial injuries among the respondents was low. However, there is a need to educate our study population on healthy social lifestyles, as well as the benefits of being compliant with road traffic regulations. Also, there exists the need to rehabilitate those with oral and facial injuries to improve their quality of life.

INTRODUCTION

Orofacial injuries can be described as injuries affecting the face, mouth structures, jaws, and orbital structures (1, 2). Orofacial injuries have various aetiological factors, and some of these factors include: road traffic accidents (RTAs); industrial trauma; falls; injuries from contact sports; and assaults (2, 3).

The incidence rate of orofacial injuries varies globally (2, 3). The incidence rates of orofacial injuries are influenced by the interplay of geographical features of an environment, social trends of the society, alcohol and drug abuse, road traffic regulations, occupation, and seasons of the year (3-13). The geographical attributes of an environment is closely related to the most prevalent aetiological factor of oral and facial injuries among the population dwelling in such places (3). For instance, the developing countries have a relatively higher number of cases of automobile crash – related oral and facial injuries when compared to the developed countries like the USA, where injuries from firearms exceeds automobile crash-related oral and facial injuries (3, 8, 14, 15). Also, when injuries in urban and rural areas were compared, it was observed that person to person violence is on the increase, resulting in the increase in the incidence of maxillofacial trauma cases in the former than in the latter (16, 17).

The incidence of oral and facial injuries is on the decrease in societies where there are strict road traffic regulations such as use of seat belts and enforcement of speed limits (17). Likewise, months of the hot season were associated with increased physical and traffic violence while increased road traffic injuries were noticed in the cold seasons (18). Furthermore, workers in some industries have been found to be at higher risks of having oral and facial injuries (19). The workers in the transportation, mining, agricultural, construction, and sport industries were found to be at higher risk due to their high risk of exposure to high velocity collision (19-22). In 2001, Feyer et al. reported that the population of workers in the transportation industry ranks third among the population at risk of work-related injuries (19).

Oral and facial injuries have different patterns of occurrence. This injury can be an isolated injury to the mouth, an isolated facial injury or a combined oral and facial injury (23-25). Among the group of isolated oral injuries, some are at higher risk of getting more traumatised than the others. For instance, the maxillary anterior teeth are the most traumatised, compared to other teeth in the mouth (25). Furthermore, there are some facial structures that are mostly affected in facial trauma. The mandible, for instance, is known to be the most commonly affected bony structure in facial injuries (26).

Oral and facial injury is a form of traumatic accidental injury (TAI) (10). Traumatic accidental injuries have generally been found to be one of the leading causes of deaths in the first four decades of life and they also cause a greater loss of working years than cancers and heart diseases (10). For those that survived severe cases of traumatic injuries, they do eventually develop complications that can reduce their quality of life (27, 28). Some of these complications include reduced self-esteem, reduced masticatory function and reduced facial aesthetics (27, 28). Oral and facial injury is a matter of public health importance because it results in negative physiological, psychological, social, and economic impact on individuals that are affected, and it affects a lot of people in the population (28).

The majority of studies on crash-related orofacial injuries in Nigeria were undertaken in the major cities while very few were in non-city areas (23, 29-31). Therefore, there is a need to determine the prevalence, pattern and psychosocial impact of orofacial injuries among the vulnerable population in rural areas in Nigeria. This study aims to determine the prevalence, pattern and psychosocial impact of orofacial injuries among commercial motorcyclists, drivers, and bus conductors in Eruwa, Lanlate, and Igboora communities of Oyo State, South-western Nigeria. The information provided from this study will help in appropriate policy making as regards the prevention and management of crash-related oral and facial injuries in these communities.

OUR STUDY

Approval to undertake the study was obtained from the Community Dentistry Unit, Faculty of Dentistry, University of Ibadan, since study was part of rural posting programme of the University. This study was a descriptive cross sectional study conducted under strict compliance with the Helsinki Declaration on human subject research. Study participants were commercial motorcyclists, drivers, and bus conductors in the Lanlate, Eruwa, and Igbo Ora communities of the Ibarapa East and Central Local Government Areas of Oyo state, Nigeria.

The minimum sample size for this study (n=126) was calculated using the Kish and Leslie formula for study population < 10,000 at a prevalence of injuries of 9.1% derived from a previous study among commercial taxi drivers (32).

Three trained dental students (authors: KKK, OAL, and ZOA) pre-tested a semi-structured questionnaire that assessed socio-demographic characteristics, social lifestyles, presence and pattern of facial injury, if present, among 20 commercial drivers and motorcyclists in Yemetu Community, a community in Ibadan, Oyo State, Nigeria. The three trained dental students interviewed the study participants with the pre-tested questionnaire. A modified and abridged version of the psychosocial impact of dental aesthetics questionnaire (PIDAQ) was used to assess psychosocial impact of oral and/or facial injury. The questionnaire was translated to Yoruba, the local language of inhabitants of the communities where the study was undertaken. Convenient sampling technique was adopted for participants' selection. Only 100 individuals volunteered to participate in this study, and they all gave verbal informed consent before being interviewed. Collected data were cleaned, coded and entered into the Statistical Package for Social Sciences (SPSS) version 16 software for statistical analysis. Frequency and means (±SD) were generated.

FINDINGS

One hundred and forty commercial motorcyclists, drivers, and bus conductors were invited to participate in the study; however only 100 (71.4%) agreed and consented to participate. All respondents were males, and their mean (±SD) age was 32.22 (±8.79) years. Seventy seven (77.0%) were married, ninety seven (97.0%) were Yorubas, 55 (55.0%) had secondary school education, and thirty six (36.0%) were commercial drivers (see Table 1).

Table 1. Socio-demographic characteristics of respondents (n=100)

Socio-demographic characteristics	**N**	%***
Gender		
Male	100	100.0
Female	0	0.0
Mean (±SD)** age* years	32.22 (±8.79)	
Marital status		
Single	23	23.0
Married	77	77.0
Tribe		
Yoruba	97	97.0
Others	3	3.0
Level of education		
No formal education	7	7.0
Primary	23	23.0
Secondary	55	55.0
Tertiary	15	15.0
Occupation		
Driver	36	36.0
Motorcyclist	62	62.0
Conductor	2	2.0

*Age in years; **SD = Standard deviation; ***percentages were calculated based the total number of respondents; n = total number of respondents; N = total number of respondents in each category.

Less than half (42.0%) of the respondents had never consumed alcohol, while only 24.0% consumed alcohol on daily basis. Furthermore, the majority (90%) of the respondents do not smoke tobacco. Only ten (10.0%) respondents gave a positive history of tobacco smoking; of which all of them reported that they smoke tobacco everyday (see Table 2).

Of the 36 commercial drivers that participated in this study, only 72.2% of them reported to use seat belt always, when driving (see Table 3). Only three (4.8%) of the 62 commercial motorcyclists reported to wear helmet when riding a motorcycle while 31 (50%) had never worn it when riding a motorcycle (see Table 4). Also, none of the two participating bus conductors had ever used seat belt when on highway (see Table 5).

Table 2. Frequency of alcohol and tobacco consumption among respondents (n=100)

Frequency of consumption	Alcohol N (%)	Tobacco N (%)
Never	42 (42)	90 (90)
Daily	24 (24)	10 (10)
Weekly	25 (25)	0 (0)
Monthly	9 (9)	0 (0)

N = total number of respondents in each category.

Table 3. Frequency of use of seat belts among those respondents that were commercial drivers

Frequency (n=36)	N	%*
Never	3	8.3
Rare	2	5.6
Sometimes	5	13.9
Always	26	72.2

*Percentages were calculated based on the total number of respondents that were commercial drivers; n = total number of respondents that were commercial drivers; N = total number of respondents in each category.

Table 4. Frequency of use of crash helmets among the respondents that were commercial motorcyclists

Frequency (n=62)	N	%
Never	31	50.0
Rare	9	14.5
Sometimes	19	30.6
Always	3	4.8

*Percentages were calculated based on the total number of respondents that were commercial motorcyclists; n = total number of respondents that were commercial motorcyclists; N = total number of respondents in each category.

Only 5 (13.9%) and 3 (8.3%), out of all the participating commercial motorcyclists and drivers respectively, had a positive history of automobile crash-related injury to oral structures (see Table 6). However, only 2 (5.6%) of the commercial drivers and 3 (4.8%) of the motorcyclists had a positive history of automobile crash-related facial injury (see Table 7).

Table 5. Frequency of use of crash helmets among the respondents that were bus conductors

Frequency (n=2)	**N**	%*
Never	2	100.0
Rare	0	0.0
Sometimes	0	0.0
Always	0	0.0

*Percentages were calculated based on the total number of respondents that were bus conductors; n = total number of respondents that were bus conductors; N = total number of respondents in each category.

Table 6. Comparison between occupations of respondents with exposure to automobile crash-related oral injury

	Have you ever had any automobile crash-related injury affecting your mouth since the day you have started your occupation as a driver/motorcyclist/conductor?			
Occupation		Yes (%)*	No (%)*	p – value (X^2)
	Driver	3 (8.3)	33 (91.7)	0.914
	Motorcyclist	5 (13.9)	57 (86.1)	
	Conductor	0 (0.0)	2 (100.0)	

*Percentages were calculated based on the total number of respondents in each occupational category (36 drivers, 62 motorcyclists, 2 conductors).

Table 7. Comparison between occupations of respondents with exposure to automobile crash-related facial injury

	Have you ever had any automobile crash-related injury affecting your face since the day you have started your occupation as a driver/motorcyclist/conductor?			
Occupation		Yes (%)*	No (%)*	p – value (X^2)
	Driver	2 (5.6)	34 (94.4)	0.936
	Motorcyclist	3 (4.8)	59 (95.2)	
	Conductor	0 (0.0)	2 (2.0)	

*Percentages were calculated based on the total number of respondents in each occupational category (36 drivers, 62 motorcyclists, 2 conductors).

Figure 1 shows the pattern of orofacial injuries among the respondents. Six (6.0%) respondents sustained injury to their anterior teeth, while 5 (5.0%) gave sustained injury to the temporal region of their head.

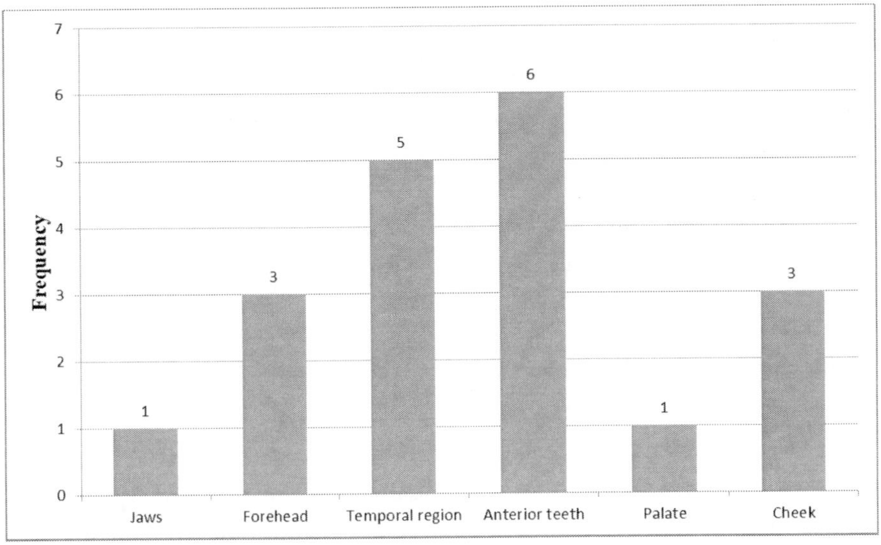

Figure 1. Pattern and frequency distribution of orofacial injuries among the respondents.

Table 8. Psychosocial impact of oral and facial appearance on respondents with histories of crash-related oral and facial injuries

Psychological statements	**Structures affected**			
	Face (N=5)		Oral cavity (N=8)	
	Yes No. (%)	No No. (%)	Yes No. (%)	No (No. (%)
I am pleased with the appearance of my face and/or teeth	5 (100.0)	0 (0.0)	7 (87.5)	1 (12.5)
I like to show off with my face and/or teeth whenever I smile	4 (80.0)	1 (20.0)	5 (62.5)	3 (37.5)
Sometimes I feel people are staring at my face and/or teeth for some anomaly	1 (20.0)	4 (80.0)	3 (37.5)	5 (62.5)
I wish my teeth and/or face looks better	3 (60.0)	2 (40.0)	6 (75.0)	2 (25.0)
I do not like checking my teeth and/or face in the mirror	2 (40.0)	3 (60.0)	7 (87.5)	1 (12.5)

N = total number of respondents in each category.

Table 8 shows the impact of automobile crash-related orofacial injuries on the psychosocial wellbeing of the respondents with history of such injury. A higher proportion of the respondents with history of facial injury were pleased with their orofacial appearance, and not suspicious of other people staring at their orofacial appearance, when compared with those with history of oral injury. A higher proportion of those with history of oral injury also wished to have better orofacial appearance, when compared to those with history of facial injury.

DISCUSSION

In this study, we undertook a survey of bus conductors, commercial motorcyclists and drivers in Eruwa, Lanlate, and Igboora communities of Oyo State, Nigeria. These three communities have a total number of four major commercial motor parks with some other minor motor parks, as at the time of data collection process. The minor motor parks were located within the campuses of the higher institutions situated within these three communities. The major motor parks were not located within any educational facility, they were social facilities provided by the government for the general public. Their upkeep and day-to-day management is under the control of the National Union of Road Transport Workers (NURTW), a trade union of commercial road transporters. People visit these busy major parks to travel out of these communities. Also, these parks serve as the final terminus of commercial buses and cars carrying goods and people into these communities.

It is noteworthy that all the respondents in this study were males as in other previous studies (33, 34). Male dominance in the transportation industry in Nigeria can be because the transportation job is generally perceived in Nigeria to be men's work. The mean (±SD) age of the respondents was 32.22 (±8.79) years. Similar age distribution had also been reported in other Nigerian studies (31, 33-35).

The majority of the respondents in this study were Yorubas, indicating a skewed tribal distribution among the commercial transporters in the Ibarapa communities. This may be attributed to the rural setting of our study location, unlike in the urban areas where there is more diversity.

The majority of the respondents had formal education, more than half of them had secondary school education indicating that they could read and write; hence they would have less difficulty in reading traffic regulation guides. In a study conducted among fuel tanker drivers in Lagos, Nigeria, a similar level of formal education was reported among the majority of the respondents (33). This indicates that literates are many among commercial transporters in Nigeria.

The social lifestyles of people vary with occupation and geography (36, 37). It has been documented that prevalence of alcoholism is higher among the non-white collar job workers, compared to white collar job workers (37); the commercial drivers, commercial motorcyclists, and bus conductors fall under the population of non-white collar workers. Some Nigerian studies had repeatedly documented a high prevalence of alcoholism (>66.0%) among commercial transporters (33, 38, 39). The findings from these studies corroborate with ours, as a significantly high proportion (58.0%) of our respondents were found to be alcoholics.

Tobacco consumption has been found to vary across age groups, gender, and occupation (40). Workers in the transportation industry ranked third among the occupational groups with the highest prevalence of tobacco consumption (40).

However, in this study, we obtained a prevalence rate of 10% on tobacco consumption among our respondents. This prevalence rate is similar to that reported by Usman & Ipinmoye (34), in a study they conducted among a group of commercial drivers in the city of Akure, Nigeria.

Non-compliance with traffic regulations had been proven to be strongly associated with automobile crashes (17). The incidence of crash-related oral and facial injuries is on the decrease in societies where there are strict road traffic regulations (17). Some of the major road traffic regulations include the appropriate use of seat belts while driving, the appropriate use of crash helmets while riding bikes, avoidance of alcohol and tobacco consumption before and during driving/riding, and avoidance of excessive speed (17). Unfortunately, a significant proportion of our respondents were not complaint with the traffic regulations, as some of them ply the roads without the use of safety belts/crash helmets. In fact, some of them consume alcohol on daily basis; this will invariably affect their level of concentration while at work. These harmful driving/riding behaviours are highly prevalent causes of automobile crashes in the Nigerian society (33, 34).

However, the prevalence of automobile crash-related orofacial injuries is relatively low among our respondents (see Tables 6 & 7); this prevalence rate is very low when compared to that reported in the urban and semi-urban places in Nigeria (22, 31). This relatively low prevalence in our study area may be attributed to reduced traffic congestions in the rural areas when compared with the urban areas.

In this present study, a higher proportion of the commercial motorcyclists reported to have sustained automobile crash-related orofacial injuries, when compared with the drivers. This may be because of the higher risk of sustaining injury from a bike than a bus/car. Also, our findings showed that the anterior teeth, cheek, forehead and temporal areas were the commonly affected areas in automobile crash-related injuries.

The survivors of traumatic orofacial injuries could develop posttraumatic complications that may reduce their quality of life (27, 28). Some of these complications include reduced self-esteem, reduced masticatory function and reduced facial aesthetics (27, 28). Based on our findings, the respondents with histories of crash-related oral injuries had a reduced quality of psychosocial life, compared to those that had facial injuries. For example, the majority of the respondents who had injuries affecting their oral structures reported that they wish that they have better aesthetic appearance when compared with those who had injuries to their face.

However, this study has its limitations. This study may not give the exact picture of the prevalence of alcoholism and tobacco consumption among our study population, as we could not ascertain the validity and reliability of their declarations on alcohol and tobacco consumption. Also, alcoholism, smoking, and non-use of seat belts and/or crash helmets are not the only predisposing factors to automobile crash-related injuries; this study did not assess other potential risk factors such as visual acuity, quality of roads, and the enforcements of road traffic regulations in these communities. Also, there are many factors that could affect the orofacial aesthetic appearance of an individual. Only the association between histories of automobile crash-related orofacial injuries with the psychosocial satisfaction of respondents' orofacial appearance was investigated in this study; other influencing factors on aesthetic appearance were not explored in this present study.

The authors recommend that the commercial motorcyclists, bus conductors, and drivers in Ibarapa Land should be educated on the benefits of compliance with road traffic regulations. They also need to be educated on the adverse medical effects of alcohol and tobacco consumption especially when driving/riding. Educating them on the benefits of the use of safety belts and crash helmets will also help in reducing the incidence of crash injuries among them. Strict traffic regulations need to be enforced on all users of highways in these communities, as many of our study respondents were noncompliant with road traffic regulations. Lastly, we recommend that those affected with orofacial injuries should be given rehabilitative treatment.

CONCLUSION

The majority of the study respondents consume alcohol; however only few of them take tobacco. Many of them were not compliant with road traffic regulations. The prevalence of oral and facial injuries among the respondents was 8% and 5% respectively. Oral injury tends to negatively affect its victims psychosocially when compared to facial injuries. There exists the need to educate our study population on the harmful effect of tobacco and alcohol consumption as well as the dangers and benefits of compliance with road traffic regulations. Also, there exists the need to rehabilitate those with oral and facial injuries for them to have a better quality of life.

ACKNOWLEDGMENTS

This study was extracted from the undergraduate student thesis of KKK, OAL, and ZOA. Authors deeply express their sincere gratitude to OI for the supervision and in-depth review of this research and manuscript. Authors appreciate the participants for taking part in the study. Authors also appreciate the traditional rulers and government authorities of the surveyed communities for giving their consent to carry out this study. The abstract of this paper was presented at the 2016 Postgraduate Conference of the Faculty of Dentistry, University of Ibadan, Nigeria. The authors have no competing interest to declare.

REFERENCES

[1] Oral & Maxillofacial Associates (OMA). Facial injuries and trauma. URL: www.omaok.com/index.asp?N=oral-surgeon-Oklahoma-City-OK-Facial-Injuries-Trauma&C=739&P=13367.

[2] Adeyemo WL, Ladeinde AL, Ogunlewe MO, James O. Trends and characteristics of oral and maxillofacial injuries in Nigeria: a review of the literature. Head Face Med 2005:1:7 doi:10.1186/1746-160X-1-7.

[3] Lee K. Global trends in maxillofacial fractures. Craniomaxillofac Trauma Reconstruction 2012;5(4):213-222.

[4] Singaram M, G SV, Udhayakumar RK. Prevalence, pattern, etiology, and management of maxillofacial trauma in a developing country: a retrospective study. J Korean Assoc Oral Maxillofac Surg 2016;42(4):174-81.

[5] Muraoka M, Nakai Y. Twenty years of statistics and observation of facial bone fracture. Acta Otolaryngol Suppl 1998;538:261-5.

[6] Montovani JC, de Campos LM, Gomes MA, de Moraes VR, Ferreira FD, Nogueira EA. Etiology and incidence of facial fractures in children and adults. Braz J Otorhinolaryngol 2006;72(2):235-41.

[7] Ashar A, Khateery S, Kovacs A. Etiology and patterns of facial fractures in Al-Ain, United Arab Emirates. Saudi Dent J 1999;11:109-13.

[8] Ugboko V, Udoye C, Ndukwe K,Amole A, Aregbesola S. Zygomatic complex fractures in a suburban Nigerian population. Dent Traumatol 2005;21(2):70-5.

[9] Zargar M, Khaji A, Karbakhsh M, Zarei MR. Epidemiology study of facial injuries during a 13 month of trauma registry in Tehran. Indian J Med Sci 2004;58(3):109-14.

[10] Gassner R, Tuli T, Hächl O, Rudisch A, Ulmer H. Cranio-maxillofacial trauma: a 10-year review of 9,543 cases with 21,067 injuries. J Craniomaxillofac Surg 2003;31(1):51-61.

[11] Maladiere E, Bado F, Meningaud JP, Guilbert F, Bertrand JC. Aetiology and incidence of facial fractures sustained during sports: a prospective study of 140 patients. Int J Oral Maxillofac Surg 2001;30(4):291-5.

[12] Hogg NJ, Stewart TC, Armstrong JE, Girotti MJ. Epidemiology of maxillofacial injuries at trauma hospitals in Ontario, Canada, between 1992 and 1997. J Trauma 2000;49(3):425-32.

[13] Sinclair JH. The changing pattern of maxilla-facial injuries. Ann R Australas Coll Dent Surg 1979;6:43-9.

[14] Champion HR, Rob CG, Trunkey DD. Foreword. In: Ryan JM, Dale RF, Morgans BT, Cooper GJ, eds. Ballistic trauma. London: Arnold, 1997.

[15] Perkins CS, Layton SA. The aetiology of maxillofacial injuries and the seat belt law. Br J Oral Surg 1998;26:353-63.

[16] Telfer MR, Jones GM, Shepherd JP. Trends in the aetiology of maxillofacial fractures in the United Kingdom. Br J Oral Maxillofac Surg 1991;29(4):250-5.

[17] Simpson DA, McLean AJ. Epidemiology. In: Simpson DA, David D, eds. Craniomaxillofacial trauma. London: Churchill Livingstone, 1995;85-99.

[18] Van Hoof RF, Merkx CA, Stekelenberg EC. The different patterns of fractures of the facial skeleton in four European countries. Int J Oral Surg 1977;6:3-11.

[19] Feyer AM, Williamson AM, Stout N, Driscoll T, Usher H, Langley JD. Comparison of work related injuries in the United States, Australia, and New Zealand: Method and overall findings. Inj Prev 2001;7:22-8.

[20] Bailer AJ, Bena JF, Stayner LT, Halperin WE, Park RM. External cause-specific summaries of occupational fatal injuries. Part II: An analysis of years of potential life lost. Am J Industr Med 2003;43:251-61.

[21] Richardson D, Loomis D, Wolf SH, Gregory E. Fatal Agricultural Injuries in North Carolina by Race and Occupation, 1977-1991. Am J Ind Med 1997;31:452-8.

[22] Fasola AO, Lawoyin JO, Obiechina AE, Arotiba JT. Inner city maxillofacial fractures due to road traffic accidents. Dent Traumatol 2003;19(1):2-5.

[23] Ogundare BO, Bonnick A, Bayley N. Pattern of mandibular fractures in an urban major trauma center. J Oral Maxillofac Surg 2003;61(6):713-8.

[24] Igboko VI, Odusanya SA, Fagade OO. Maxillofacial fractures in a semi-urban Nigerian teaching hospital. A review of 442 cases. Int J Oral Maxillofac Surg 1998;27(4):286-9.

[25] Andreasen JO. Traumatic dental injuries: A manual, 2nd edition. Oxford: Blackwell, 2003.

[26] Zachariades N, Mezitis M, Mourouzis C, Papadakis D, Spanou A. Fractures of the mandibular condyle: a review of 466 cases. Literature review, reflections on treatment and proposals. J Craniomaxillofac Surg 2006;34(7):421-32.

[27] Levine E, Degutis L, Pruzinsky T, Shin J, Persing JA. Quality of life and facial trauma: psychological and body image effects. Ann Plast Surg 2005;54(5):502-10.

[28] Kendrick D, O'Brien C, Christie N, Coupland C, Quinn C, Avis M, et al. The impact of injuries study. multicentre study assessing physical, psychosocial, social and occupational functioning post injury: A protocol. BMC Public Health 2011:11:963. doi: 10.1186/1471-1471-2458-11-963.

[29] Adekeye EO. The pattern of fractures of the facial skeleton in Kaduna, Nigeria: a survey of 1447 cases. Oral Surg Oral Med Oral Pathol 1980; 49:491.

[30] Adebayo ET, Ajike OS, Adekeye EO. Analysis of pattern of maxillofacial fractures in Kaduna, Nigeria. Br J Oral Maxillofac Surg 2003;41(6):396-400.

[31] Akhigbe OP. Motorcycle related maxillofacial injuries in a semi-urban town in Nigeria: a four year review of cases in Irrua Specialist Teaching Hospital. Dissertation. Umea: Umea International School of Public Health, 2010.

[32] Barbosa KG, Lucas-Neto A, Gama BD, Lima-Neto JC, Lucas RS, d'Avila S. Injuries and absenteeism among motorcycle taxi drivers who are victims of road traffic accidents. J Forensic Leg Med 2014;26C:15-8.

[33] Makanjuola AB, Aina OF, Onigbogi L. Alcohol and other psychoactive substance use among tanker drivers in Lagos, Nigeria. Eur Sci J 2014;10(15);545-59.

[34] Usman SO, Ipinmoye TO. Use of cigarette and marijuana among long distance commercial drivers in Akure, Ondo State, Nigeria. Eur J Forensic Sci 2016;3(1):1-4.

[35] Obuekwe ON, Ojo MA, Akpata O, Etetafia M. Maxillofacial trauma due to road traffic accidents in Benin City, Nigeria: A prospective study. Anna Afr Med 2003;2(2):58-63.

[36] Kissim B, Begleiter H. eds. The biology of alcoholism: Social aspects of alcoholism. New York: Plenum Press, 1972.

[37] Olkinuora M. Alcoholism and occupation. Scand J Work Environ Health 1984;10(6 Spec No):511-5.

[38] Bello S, Ndifon WO, Mpama EA, Oduwole OO. Pattern of alcohol use among drivers of commercial vehicles in Calabar. East Afr Med J 2011;88(3):75-9.

[39] Ogazi C, Edison E. The drink driving situation in Nigeria. Traffic Inj Prev 2012;13(2):115-9.

[40] Centre for Disease Control and Prevention. Current cigarette smoking prevalence among working adults – United States, 2004-2010. MMWR 2011;60(38):1305-9.

In: Disability: International Aspects
Editors: Ariel Tenenbaum et al.
ISBN: 978-1-53617-886-9

Chapter 13

CUT OFF SCORE OF FIVE TIMES SIT-TO-STAND TEST TO PREDICT RISK OF FALLS IN THAI COMMUNITY-DWELLING OLDER ADULTS

Puttipong Poncumhak*[1,*]*, MSc, PT,
Arunrat Srithawong*[1]*, MSc, PT
and Winut Duangsanjun*[2]*, MNS, RN
[1]Department of Physical Therapy, School of Allied Health Sciences, University of Phayao, Phayao
[2]Adult and Gerontological Nursing, Faculty of Nursing, Vongchavalitkul University, Nakhon Ratchasima Province, Thailand

ABSTRACT

* Corresponding Author: Assistant professor Puttipong Poncumhak, MSc, PT, School of Allied Health Sciences, University of Phayao, Phayao, Thailand 56000. E-mail: puttipong.po@up.ac.th.

In this chapter we aimed to determine the specific cut-off score for the five times sit-to-stand test (FTSST) to predict the risk of falling among Thai community-dwelling elderly by decade of age and gender. A total of 387 participants aged 60 years and older, with and without a history of falling, were assessed for their functional ability using the FTSST. The results of the study showed that the average time recorded for the FTSST was significantly different for the three decades assessed ($p < 0.001$). The participants in the faller group required significantly more time to complete the test than did those in the non-faller group ($p < 0.001$). In all decades, the females took significantly longer to complete the FTSST than the males ($p < 0.05$). The results provided an optimal cut-off score for the FTSST in each gender group by decade in the range of 11.01–14.43 seconds, with high sensitivity and specificity and good-to-excellent AUC values. The findings of the study identified optimal cut-off scores for each age and gender group for reliable fall-risk prediction in Thai community-dwelling elderly.

INTRODUCTION

It is acknowledged that advanced age is associated with physiological changes in many body systems, especially in those aged 75 years and older (1). A literature review indicates that musculoskeletal decline in elderly likely relates to a decrease in muscle mass, bone mass density and muscle strength (2, 3). The loss of muscle mass associated with the presence of low muscle function (strength or physical performance) is one of the main causes of mobility loss and disability related to ageing (4). Deficiencies in mobility, self-care and self-management result in an increased risk for older adults of falling and the consequences of falls, such as fractures, loss of confidence, the burden of care by others (5) and increased re-hospitalisation and mortality rates (5-7). Falls are the primary cause of the loss of independent living and the development of fear, which may result in severe limitations to physical activity, a loss of social contact and even death (8, 9). More than one in three people a year over 65 years of age experience a fall and in half of these cases, falls are recurrent (10). About 10% of elderly who fall experience serious results (10, 11) and are admitted to emergency departments, leading to hospitalisation (12). Moreover, falls account for the largest percentage of deaths in the elderly

(13). Therefore, it is vital to develop a fall-risk assessment tool that measures muscle strength and that can be used as an objective and standard tool.

The five times sit-to-stand test (FTSST) is a commonly used test for measuring functional lower extremities muscle strength (7). The test directly records performance and provides objective data that allow outcomes to be compared between testers and test intervals. Furthermore, the test is not complex, does not require costly equipment and can be easily administered to larger populations (14, 15). In addition, the FTSST can be used as a functional tool to assess muscle strength in many populations, such as spinal cord injury patients (16), stroke patients (17) and the elderly (7, 8, 15, 18, 19). The FTSST has been used to test psychometric properties in the elderly, finding a correlation between force and the torque of knee extensors ($r = -0.48$ to -0.57) (20). In addition, the FTSST has convergent validity with the timed up and go test (TUGT) ($r = 0.73$) and walking speed ($r = -0.82$) (21). Moreover, the test has been found to have predictive validity to predict the risk of falls in the elderly; those who took more than 15 seconds to perform the test were found to have a high risk of falls (22).

A review analysis demonstrated that individuals with times for five repetitions of this test exceeding the following can be considered to have worse than average performance: 11.4 sec (60 to 69 years), 12.6 sec (70 to 79 years) and 14.8 sec (80 to 89 years) (7). Although some studies have reported cut-off points for the FTSST to predict falls in elderly Thai people (15), the findings did not divide the elderly into groups according to their decade of age, which may affect their physical ability. Therefore, this study aimed to explore the outcome of the FTSST and specific cut-off scores for the FTSST to predict falls in Thai community-dwelling elderly according to their decade of age and gender.

OUR STUDY

The cross-sectional study recruited both male and female participants aged 60 years and older dwelling in the community. There were 129 participants per group, the sample size being calculated for adequate sensitivity/specificity. The 387 participants were divided into three groups (129 per group) according to decade of age: young-old (60–69 years), middle-old (70–79 years) and oldest-old (80 years and over). The participants were included if they were able to stand up from a chair or bed independently without using hands or assistive devices, and were alert and oriented. Exclusionary criteria were based on severe underlying diseases that might affect the outcome of the study, significant pain in the lower extremities of more than 5 of 10 on a visual analogue scale, active infection or diagnosis of cancer, current injury, uncorrected visual deficits and amputation of an extremity. The study was approved by the Clinical Research Ethics Committee of the University of Phayao, Phayao, Thailand (Ethics Committee reference number: 2/094/59), which requires informed consent to be obtained.

Procedures

The participants were interviewed and assessed for their eligibility according to the criteria of the study and demographic data, including age, gender, height, weight, underlying diseases and fall history over the preceding six months, using a questionnaire. In addition, participants were evaluated for the FTSST. Details of the FTSST are explained below.

The five times sit-to-stand test (FTSST)

The participants were required to sit on a standard armless chair with back upright and hip flexion of 90 degrees, with their feet placed flat on the floor at 10 cm behind the knees, and with their arms on their sides. Then the subjects were instructed to stand up with the hips and knees in full extension, and sit down five times at the fastest safe speed without using the arms. The time required to complete the test was recorded by performed three trials, with a period of rest as needed between the trials.

Then the average findings of the three trials were used for data analyses. During the test, subjects did not wear shoes, in order to prevent shoe type variation affecting the outcome. In addition, the subjects had to wear a lightweight safety belt around their waist, with a physiotherapist walking or being alongside the subjects throughout the tests in order to ensure the subjects' safety and improve the accuracy of the outcome. (8, 15).

Statistical analysis

The data analysis was performed using STATA/SE 14.1 for Windows (StataCorp LP, 4905 Lakeway Drive College Station, TX 77845, USA). Descriptive statistics were applied to explain the baseline demographics and findings of the study. A one-way analysis of variance (one-way ANOVA) was applied to compare outcomes of the FTSST, BMI and age groups, and a post hoc analysis (Scheffé test) was used to identify the differences in every pairwise condition. The outcomes of the FTSST between fallers and non-fallers were compared by use of the independent sample t-test. Receiver-operating characteristic (ROC) curves were utilised to explore an optimal cut-off score, sensitivity, specificity, accuracy and area under the ROC curve (AUC) for the FTSST to indicate fall risk. The level of significance was set at $p < 0.05$.

Table 1. Demographics data of participants (n = 128 participants/group)

Variables	Young old	Middle old	Oldest old
Age*: years (maen ± SD)	64.36 ± 2.43	73.78 ± 2.71	83.52±3.71
Gender: n (%)			
Male	58 (44.96)	56 (43.41)	68 (52.71)
Female	71 (55.04)	73 (56.59)	71 (47.29)
BMI: kg/m^2 (mean±SD)	23.18 ± 3.10	22.94 ± 3.00	23.05±3.34
History of fall: n (%)			
non-faller	81 (62.79)	69 (53.49)	70 (54.26)
faller	48 (37.21)	60 (46.51)	59 (45.74)
FTSST*: s (mean±SD)	10.29 ± 2.48	12.30 ± 3.25	14.22 ± 4.32

Note: *p-value from one-way ANOVA and post hoc analysis $p < 0.001$.
n; number, SD; standard deviation, BMI; body mass index, FTSST; five times sit-to-stand test.

Table 2. Comparison of outcome of FTSST between fall history group according to decade of age

Age decade	Faller (s)	Non-faller (s)	P value*
Young old	11.98 ± 1.16	9.29 ± 2.10	<0.001
Middle old	14.51 ± 2.87	10.39 ± 2.16	<0.001
Oldest old	16.67 ± 4.17	11.30 ± 2.17	<0.001

Note: *P value from independent sample t test. s; seconds.

FINDINGS

The baseline demographics and the mean time to complete the FTSST of subjects according to age decade are shown in Table 1. Most of the subjects were female. The results of the study showed that the average time to complete the FTSST was significantly different in all three age groups ($p < 0.001$). In each age group, subjects in the faller group required significantly more time to complete the tests than those in the non-faller group ($p < 0.001$) (see Table 2). Table 3 shows that female subjects took significantly longer to complete the FTSST male subjects in all age groups ($p < 0.05$). Tables 4 and 5 shows the optimal cut-off scores, sensitivity, specificity, accuracy and AUC for the FTSST according to decade of age and gender.

Table 3. Comparison of outcome of FTSST between male and female according to decade of age

Age decade	Male (s)	Female (s)	P value
Young old	9.83 ± 2.24	11.67 ± 2.62	<0.05
Middle old	11.93 ± 2.76	13.79 ± 3.76	<0.05
Oldest old	13.17 ± 3.52	15.07 ± 4.74	<0.05

Note: *P value from independent sample t test. s; seconds.

Table 4. The optimal cut off score, sensitivity, specificity, accuracy, and AUC of the FTSST according to decade of age

Age decade	Cut off (s)	Sensitivity (%)	Specificity (%)	Accuracy (%)	AUC (95%CI)
Young old	11.01	77.08	76.54	74.42	0.832 (0.762-0.901)
Middle old	12.14	83.33	86.96	83.72	0.904 (0.852-0.955)
Oldest old	13.00	80.00	79.66	75.97	0.901 (0.851-0.950)

Note: AUC; area under ROC curve, CI; confident interval, s; seconds.

Table 5. The optimal cut off score, sensitivity, specificity, accuracy, and AUC of the FTSST according to decade of age and gender

Age decade	Gender	Cut off (s)	Sensitivity (%)	Specificity (%)	Accuracy (%)	AUC (95%CI)
Young old	Male	11.01	70.59	82.93	75.86	0.827 (0.716-0.939)
	Female	11.05	80.65	70.00	73.24	0.818 (0.720-0.917)
Middle old	Male	12.60	92.31	93.33	89.29	0.961 (0.918-1.00)
	Female	12.14	76.47	82.05	76.71	0.864 (0.780-0.948)
Oldest old	Male	13.69	72.41	86.21	79.31	0.904 (0.830-0.976)
	Female	14.43	70.73	76.67	71.83	0.892 (0.821-0.964)

Note: AUC; area under ROC curve, CI; confident interval, s; seconds.

DISCUSSION

Muscle mass loss has a cause-effect relationship with muscle strength. Loss of both muscle mass and strength increase with age and is a problem for the elderly since it can result in a poor quality of life and physical disabilities (23). Moreover, muscle strength is a strong predictor of severe mobility limitation, slow gait speed, increased fall risk, risk of hospitalisation and high mortality rate (24). For example, older adults with low muscle strength have a 2.6-fold greater risk of severe mobility limitation, 4.3-fold greater risk of slow gait speed, and 2.1-fold greater risk of mortality compared to older adults with high muscle strength (25). The FTSST is a commonly used standard functional tool to measure muscle strength. Moreover, it has been applied as a screening tool for falls (15, 19). The present study confirms the ability of the FTSST to assess clearly the lower extremities muscle strength of the elderly according decade of age ($p < 0.001$, see Table 1). In addition, significant differences were found between subjects who were fallers and those who were non-fallers ($P < 0.001$, see Table 2).

When considering gender differentiation, the present study showed that females took a significantly longer time to complete the FTSST than did males in all age decades ($p < 0.05$, see Table 3). This shows that gender affects the ability to perform the FTSST. Thaweewannakij and colleagues reported that the lower extremities muscle strength of Thai male participants were significantly better than those of female participants in the middle-old and oldest-old ($p < 0.01$), except in those who were 60 to 69 years of age ($P > .05$)(26). The findings of the present study and that previous study may be due to the differences in size and number of muscle fibres between males and females. A previous study confirmed that females had 30% and 25% smaller cross-sectional muscle areas for the vastus lateralis and total knee extensors, respectively, than men ($p < 0.01$) (27). The results indicate that the primary determinant of the greater muscle strength of males is their larger mean fibre areas, which result in greater cross-sectional muscle areas. In addition, a study by Miller et al. (27) reported that males had significantly larger type II fibre areas and mean fibre areas in the vastus lateralis than women did ($p < 0.05$) (27).

An ROC curve is a plot of sensitivity against 1- specificity and measures a test's performance. The better the test, the closer the ROC curve approaches the top left-hand corner, which represents the combination of 100% sensitivity and 100% specificity (28). Sensitivity and specificity, the former defined as the number of true positive decisions/the number of actually positive cases, and the latter defined as the number of true negative decisions/the number of actually negative cases, constitute the basic measures of performance of diagnostic tests (29). A test that perfectly discriminates between subjects who fall and non-fall would yield a curve that coincides with the left and top side of the plot. In addition, a perfect test would have an AUC of 1.0, while a completely useless test would have an AUC of 0.5. In other words, the closer the AUC is to 1, the better the overall diagnostic performance of the test, and the closer it is to 0.5, the poorer the diagnostic performance of the test (30, 31). Hosmer and Lemeshow have provided the following classification system for the AUC: $0.7 \leq AUC < 0.8$ = "Acceptable discrimination"; $0.8 \leq AUC < 0.9$ = "Excellent discrimination"; $AUC \geq 0.9$ = "Outstanding discrimination" (32). In the present study, the cut-off score of the FTSST is in the range of 11.01–14.43 seconds, with high sensitivity and specificity and good-to-excellent AUC values when separated by age and gender. The cut-off scores in each age and gender group from this study can act as the optimal cut-off scores for reliable fall-risk prediction for the elderly. In addition, the findings of this study are consistent with the data of a previous study that reported cut-off scores for the FTSST to predict the risk of falls in the elderly according to decade of age. The data from that study showed cut-off scores of 11.4 sec (60 to 69 years), 12.6 sec (70 to 79 years) and 14.8 sec (80 to 89 years) (7). However, the data may not be used for Thai elderly because there are differences in many factors, such as physiological structure. Some studies of Thai elderly provide optimal cut-off scores for predicting the risk of falls (15, 33). One study investigated the ability of the FTSST in those aged 60 and over and provided a cut-off score for the FTSST of ≥ 10.02 sec (sensitivity 68.57%, specificity 80.00%, AUC 0.82; 95%CI = 1.32–2.58) (15). However, the mean age fell into that of the young-old and the findings did not divide the elderly groups according to decade of age and gender, factors that may affect physical ability. Moreover, previous studies have shown lower sensitivity than the present study. Therefore, the current study confirms the usefulness of the FTSST as a simple screening tool to predict risk of falls in all age decades of community-dwelling Thai elderly. The results of this study may have a significant impact on primary care clinical practice in the field of fall-risk evaluation. Physical therapists and other healthcare professionals could easily classify elderly community-dwelling subjects by fall-risk group, facilitating more effective management of fall-prevention programmes.

The conclusion of the study confirms the importance and benefits of the FTSST as a simple screening tool to predict the risk of falls in all age ranges of the elderly (33). This study provides an optimal cut-off score of the FTSST in the range of 11.01–14.43 seconds with high sensitivity and specificity and good-to-excellent AUC values according to age decade and gender.

ACKNOWLEDGMENTS

This study was financially supported by University of Phayao (Funding No. RD61077).

REFERENCES

[1] Arnau A, Espaulella J, Serrarols M, Canudas J, Formiga F, Ferrer M. Risk factors for functional decline in a population aged 75 years and older without total dependence: A one-year follow-up. Arch Gerontol Geriatr 2016;65:239-47.

[2] Helbostad JL, Sturnieks DL, Menant J, Delbaere K, Lord SR, Pijnappels M. Consequences of lower extremity and trunk muscle fatigue on balance and functional tasks in older people: a systematic literature review. BMC Geriatrics 2010;10:56.

[3] Sturnieks DL, St George R, Lord SR. Balance disorders in the elderly. Neurophysiol Clin 2008;38(6):467-78.

[4] Janssen I, Heymsfield SB, Ross R. Low relative skeletal muscle mass (sarcopenia) in older persons is associated with functional impairment and physical disability. J Am Geriatr Soc 2002;50(5):889-96.

[5] Colon-Emeric CS, Whitson HE, Pavon J, Hoenig H. Functional decline in older adults. Am Fam Physician 2013;88(6):388-94.

[6] Amarya S, Singh K, Sabharwal M. Changes during aging and their association with malnutrition. J Clin Gerontol Geriatr 2015;6(3):78-84.

[7] Bohannon RW. Reference values for the five-repetition sit-to-stand test: a descriptive meta-analysis of data from elders. Percept Mot Skills 2006;103(1):215-22.

[8] Poncumhak P, Sittitan M, Srithawong A. The development of simple screening tool for predict risk of falls in Thai community-dwelling elderly. J Med Assoc Thai 2016;99(8):7.

[9] Renfro MO, Fehrer S. Multifactorial screening for fall risk in community-dwelling older adults in the primary care office: development of the fall risk assessment & screening tool. J Geriatr Phys Ther 2011;34(4):174-83.

[10] Tinetti ME, Speechley M, Ginter SF. Risk factors for falls among elderly persons living in the community. N Eng J Med 1988;319(26):1701-7.

[11] Tinetti ME, Kumar C. The patient who falls: "It's always a trade-off". JAMA 2010;303(3):258-66.

[12] Rau CS, Lin TS, Wu SC, Yang JC, Hsu SY, Cho TY, et al. Geriatric hospitalizations in fall-related injuries. Scand J Trauma Resusc Emerg Med 2014;22:63.

[13] Burns E, Kakara R. Deaths from falls among persons aged ≥65 Years - United States, 2007-2016. MMWR 2018;67(18):509-14.

[14] Batista FS, Gomes GA, Neri AL, Guariento ME, Cintra FA, Sousa Mda L, et al. Relationship between lower-limb muscle strength and frailty among elderly people. Sao Paulo Med J 2012;130(2):102-8.

[15] Poncumhak. P, Suwannakul. B, Srithawong A. Validity of five times sit to stand test for the evaluation of risk of fall in community-dwelling older adults. J Assoc Med Sci 2016;49(2):9.

[16] Poncumhak P, Saengsuwan J, Kamruecha W, Amatachaya S. Reliability and validity of three functional tests in ambulatory patients with spinal cord injury. Spinal Cord 2013;51(3):214-7.

[17] Mong Y, Teo TW, Ng SS. 5-repetition sit-to-stand test in subjects with chronic stroke: reliability and validity. Arch Phys Med Rehabil 2010;91(3):407-13.

[18] Abe T, Thiebaud RS, Loenneke JP, Ogawa M, Mitsukawa N. Association between forearm muscle thickness and age-related loss of skeletal muscle mass, handgrip and knee extension strength and walking performance in old men and women: a pilot study. Ultrasound Med Biol 2014;40(9):2069-75.

[19] Bohannon RW. Measurement of sit-to-stand among older adults. Top Geriatr Rehabil 2012;28(1):11-6.

[20] Bohannon RW, Bubela DJ, Magasi SR, Wang YC, Gershon RC. Sit-to-stand test: Performance and determinants across the age-span. Isokinet Exerc Sci 2010;18(4):235-40.

[21] Schaubert KL, Bohannon RW. Reliability and validity of three strength measures obtained from community-dwelling elderly persons. Strength Cond Res 2005;19(3):717-20.

[22] Buatois S, Miljkovic D, Manckoundia P, Gueguen R, Miget P, Vancon G, et al. Five times sit to stand test is a predictor of recurrent falls in healthy community-living subjects aged 65 and older. J Am Geriatr Soc 2008;56(8):1575-7.

[23] Cruz-Jentoft AJ, Baeyens JP, Bauer JM, Boirie Y, Cederholm T, Landi F, et al. Sarcopenia: European consensus on definition and diagnosis: Report of the European Working Group on Sarcopenia in Older People. Age Ageing 2010;39(4):412-23.

[24] Miljkovic N, Lim JY, Miljkovic I, Frontera WR. Aging of skeletal muscle fibers. Ann Rehabil Med 2015;39(2):155-62.

[25] Manini TM, Visser M, Won-Park S, Patel KV, Strotmeyer ES, Chen H, et al. Knee extension strength cutpoints for maintaining mobility. J Am Geriatr Soc 2007;55(3):451-7.

[26] Thaweewannakij T, Wilaichit S, Chuchot R, Yuenyong Y, Saengsuwan J, Siritaratiwat W, et al. Reference values of physical performance in Thai elderly people who are functioning well and dwelling in the community. Phys ther 2013;93(10):1312-20.

[27] Miller AE, MacDougall JD, Tarnopolsky MA, Sale DG. Gender differences in strength and muscle fiber characteristics. Eur J Appl Physiol 1993;66(3):254-62.

[28] Power M, Fell G, Wright M. Principles for high-quality, high-value testing. Evid Based Med 2013;18(1):5-10.

[29] Park SH, Goo JM, Jo CH. Receiver operating characteristic (ROC) curve: practical review for radiologists. Korean J Radiol 2004;5(1):11-8.

[30] Akobeng AK. Understanding diagnostic tests 3: Receiver operating characteristic curves. Acta Paediatrica 2007;96(5):644-7.

[31] Fan J, Upadhye S, Worster A. Understanding receiver operating characteristic (ROC) curves. CJEM 2006;8(1):19-20.

[32] Hosmer DW, S L. Applied logistic regression, 2nd ed. New York: Wiley, 2000.

[33] Poncumhak P, Insorn T, Prasittimet N, Manota P. The pilot study on the risk of fall prediction in Thai elderly using five times sit-to-stand test. Srinagarind Med J 2014;29(3):237-42.

In: Disability: International Aspects
Editors: Ariel Tenenbaum et al.
ISBN: 978-1-53617-886-9

Chapter 14

THE PROJECTIONS OF MONEY VALUE OF DISABILITY-ADJUSTED-LIFE-YEARS SAVED IN ZAMBIA BETWEEN 2017 AND 2030

Joses Muthuri Kirigia[1,*], PhD, MA, DIP, BEd, Rose Nabi Deborah Karimi Muthuri[2], MA, BA and Newton Gitonga Muthuri[3], BBA

[1]African Sustainable Development Research Consortium (ASDRC), Nairobi, Kenya
[2]School of Health Systems and Public Health, Faculty of Health Sciences, University of Pretoria, Pretoria, South Africa
[3]Chandaria School of Business, United States International University, Nairobi, Kenya

* Corresponding Author: Professor Joses Muthuri Kirigia, PhD, African Sustainable Development Research Consortium (ASDRC), P.O. Box 6994 00100 GPO, Nairobi, Kenya. E-mail: muthurijoses68@gmail.com.

Abstract

The specific objectives of this chapter were to estimate the money values of disability-adjusted-life-years (DALYs) lost in Zambia in 2017 and expected in 2030; and to calculate the potential money savings from DALY losses averted assuming United Nations Sustainable Development Goal 3 (SDG3) targets are attained. A variant of the net output approach (or human capital approach) is used to monetarily value DALYs lost from 163 diseases and injuries. The potential savings equals economic value of DALYs lost in 2017 minus economic value of DALY expected in 2030. In 2017, the country lost a total of 7,919,620 DALYs from all causes with an economic value of Int$32,385,080,324. Of which, 62.5% was attributed to communicable, maternal, neonatal and nutritional diseases; 31.2% to non-communicable diseases; and 6.3% to injuries. About Int$25.14 billion (77.63%) of the economic value of DALYs lost in 2017 was from SDG3 targets related diseases and transport injuries. Full attainment of the SDG3 targets 3.1, 3.2, 3.3, 3.4 and 3.6 would save the country about Int$13 billion, i.e., 16.6% of the total GDP of Zambia in 2019. Diseases and injuries inflicts a heavy burden on the health and economy of Zambia every year. There is urgent need to increase investments into strengthening of the national health system, the other systems that tackle social determinants of health, and the national health research system to boost Zambia's probability of attaining SDG3 by 2030.

Abbreviations

AARR	Average Annual Rate of Reduction
AU	African Union
CARMA	Campaign for Accelerated Reduction of Maternal Mortality
CHE	Current health expenditure per person
CMNN	Communicable, maternal, neonatal and nutritional diseases
DALY	Disability-adjusted-life-year
DNC_{2017}	Number of deaths from NCD in 2017
DMA_{2017}	Number of deaths from malaria in 2017

$DMA_{T3.3b}$	Number of deaths from malaria in 2030 if target 3.3b is achieved
DNT_{2017}	Number of deaths from NTD in 2017
$DNT_{T3.3d}$	Expected number of deaths from NTD in 2030 assuming target 3.3d is realized
DTB_{2017}	Number of deaths from TB in 2017
$DTB_{T3.3c}$	Number of deaths from TB in 2030, if target 3.3c is reached
DTI_{2017}	Number of deaths from transport injuries in 2017
$DTI_{T3.6}$	Number of deaths from transport injuries in 2030, assuming target 3.6 is achieved
DVH_{2017}	Number of deaths from VH in 2017
$DVH_{T3.3e}$	Expected number of deaths from VH in 2030, if target 3.3e is accomplished
$EVDALY_j$	Money value of DALY losses from each jth disease or injury
$EVDALY_1$	Money value of DALYs from the first disease
$EVDALY_2$	Money value of DALYs from the second disease
$EVDALY_3$	Money value of DALYs from the third disease
$EVDALY_k$	Money value of DALYs from the kth disease.
$EVDALY_{HIV2030}$	Expected money value of DALYs lost from HIV/AIDS in 2030
$EVDALY_{HIV2017}$	Money value of DALYs lost from HIV/AIDS in 2017
$EVDALY_{HIV\text{-}SAVINGS}$	Expected savings the money value of DALYs loss from HIV/AIDS premature deaths and disability averted
$EVDALY_{MD2030}$	Expected money value of DALYs lost from maternal disorders in 2030
$EVDALY_{MD2017}$	Money value of DALYs lost from maternal disorders in 2017
$EVDALY_{MAL2030}$	Expected money value of DALYs lost from malaria in 2030
$EVDALY_{MAL2017}$	Money value of DALYs lost from malaria in 2017

$EVDALY_{NCD2030}$	Expected money value of DALYs lost from NCD in 2030
$EVDALY_{NCD2017}$	Money value of DALYs lost from NCD in 2017
$EVDALY_{ND2030}$	Expected money value of DALYs lost from neonatal disorders in 2030
$EVDALY_{ND2017}$	Money value of DALYs lost from neonatal disorders in 2017
$EVDALY_{NTDD2030}$	Expected money value of DALYs lost from NTD in 2030
$EVDALY_{NTDD2017}$	Money value of DALYs lost from NTD in 2017
$EVDALY_{TB2030}$	Expected money value of DALYs lost from TB in 2030
$EVDALY_{TBD2017}$	Money value of DALYs lost from TB in 2017
$EVDALY_{TID2030}$	Expected money value of DALYs from transport injuries in 2030
$EVDALY_{TID2017}$	Money value of DALYs from transport injuries in 2017
$EVDALY_{VH2030}$	Expected money value of DALYs lost from viral hepatitis (VH) in 2030
$EVDALY_{VH2017}$	Money value of DALYs lost from VH in 2017
GDP	Gross domestic product
HALE	Health-adjusted-life-year
HDI	Human development index
$HIVD_{2017}$	Number of HIV/AIDS deaths in 2017
$HIVD_{T3.2}$	Expected number of HIV/AIDS deaths in 2030 if target 3.3a is achieved
IHME	Institute for Health Metrics and Evaluation
INJ	Injury
Int$	International dollars or purchasing power parity
MM_{2017}	Maternal mortality ratio in 2017
$MM_{T3.1}$	Expected maternal mortality ratio in 2030 supposing target 3.1 is achieved
MNCAH	Maternal, new-born, child and adolescent health
NCD	Non-communicable diseases

$NCD_{T3.4}$	Number of deaths from NCD in 2030, assuming target 3.4 is achieved
NHRS	National health research system
NN_{2017}	Neonatal mortality ratio in 2017
$NN_{T3.2}$	Expected neonatal mortality rate in 2030 assuming target 3.2 is achieved.
NTD	Neglected tropical disease
PCGDP	Zambia's per capita GDP
PYLL	Potential years of life lost
SADC	Southern African Development Community
SDG	United Nations Sustainable Development Goal
T3.1	SDG3 target 3.1 on maternal mortality ratio
T3.2	SDG3 target 3.2 on neonatal mortality rate
T3.3a	SDG3 target 3.3a on HIV deaths
T3.3b	SDG3 target 3.3b on malaria deaths
T3.3c	SDG3 target 3.3c on TB deaths
T3.3d	SDG3 target 3.3d on NTD deaths
T3.3e	SDG3 target 3.3e on VH deaths
T3.4	SDG3 target 3.4 on NCD deaths
T3.6	SDG3 target 3.6 on transport injury deaths
UN	United Nations Organization
UNDP	United Nations Development Programme
UNGA	United Nations General Assembly
UNICEF	United Nations Children's Fund
US$	United States Dollar
WHA	World Health Assembly
WHO	World Health Organization
WHO/AFRO	WHO Regional Office for Africa
YLD	Years of life lived with a disability
YLL	Years of life lost
ZEVDALY	Total money value of the DALYs lost in Zambia

INTRODUCTION

Zambia is one of the 16 Southern African Development Community (SADC) member states (1). The country has an estimated population of 18.321 million people; and a total gross domestic product (GDP) of International Dollars (Int$) 78.128 billion (2). The GDP per capita is Int$4,264, i.e., equivalent to US$ 1,426. In 2017, the human development index (HDI) for Zambia was 0.588; and the inequality-adjusted HDI was 0.388 (3).

In 2017, a total of 7,919,620 disability-adjusted-life-years (DALYs) were lost (4). Out of which, 4,951,697.95 (62.5%) DALYs were lost from communicable, maternal, neonatal and nutritional diseases (CMNN); 2,472,273.59 (31.2%) from non-communicable diseases (NCD); and 495,648.16 (6.3%) DALYs from injuries (INJ). Between 2015 and 2017, the disease burden decreased slightly by 0.18%, i.e., from 7,934,043 to 7,919,620 DALYs.

The small reduction in the burden of disease might be attributed to three systemic weaknesses. First, the sub-optimally performing national health system. Zambia's health system is made up of eight third-level hospitals, 34 second-level hospitals, 99 first-level hospitals, 1,839 health centres, and 953 health posts (5).

The health system is operated by 1,514 medical doctors; 11,666 nursing personnel; 3,141 midwifery personnel; 312 dentists; 1,159 pharmacists; 1,796 environmental occupational health and hygiene professionals; 921 medical and pathology laboratory scientists; 1,126 medical and pathology laboratory technicians; 432 physiotherapists; 415 physiotherapy technicians and assistants 415; 3,762 community health workers (6). As shown in Table 1, the Zambia's densities of medical doctors and nursing plus midwifery personnel were 16.8-fold and 3.9-fold lower than the global averages, respectively.

Table 1. Comparison of health system indicators in Zambia, the WHO African Region and the Global

Health system indicators	Zambia	WHO African Region	Global
UHC service coverage index (2015)*	56%	44%	64%
Population with household expenditures on health >10% of total household expenditure or income (%) (2015)*	0.3	10.3	11.7
Population with household expenditures on health >25% of total household expenditure or income (%) (2015)*	0.0	2,6	2.6
Density of medical doctors (per 10 000 population) (2018)*	0.9	2.8	15.1
Density of nursing and midwifery personnel (per 10 000 population (2018)*	8.9	11.0	34.8
Average of 13 International Health Regulations core capacity scores (2018)*	31	42	60
Proportion of population using safely managed drinking-water services (%) (2015)*	47 (urban)	26	71
Proportion of population using at least basic sanitation services (%) (2015)**	39 (Rural=19; Urban=54)	31 (Rural=21; Urban=45)	68
Population with basic handwashing (with soap) facilities at home % (2015**	14 (Rural=5; Urban=26)	18 (Rural=11; Urban=29)	-
Population practising open defecation (%) (2015)	15 (Rural=25; Urban=1)	22 (Rural=31; Urban=7	0 (Europe)
Proportion of population with primary reliance on clean fuels (%) (2017)**	16	17	61
Annual mean concentrations of fine particulate matter ($PM_{2.5}$) in urban areas (μg/m3) (2016)*	24.7	35.5	39.6
Population with at least some secondary education (% ages 25 years & older) (2017)***	Female=39.2%; Male=52.4%	Female=42.9%; Male=59.45% (medium human development)	Female=69%; Male=75.7% (high human development)
Literacy rate among adults (% ages 15 and older) (2017)***	83.0	74.3 (medium human development)	94.2 (high human development)
Labour force participation rate (% ages 15 years and older) (2017)***	Female=70.1%; Male=79.7%	Female=36.8%; Male=78.9% (medium human development)	Female= 55.0%; Male=75.5% (high human development)

Table 1. (Continued)

Health system indicators	Zambia	WHO African Region	Global
Perceptions of individual well-being: % who felt safe***	Female= 43; Male = 53	Female=64; Male=75	Female=61; Male=75
Prevalence of stunting in children under 5 (%) (2018)*	40	33.1	21.9
Prevalence of wasting in children under 5 (%) (2018)*	6.2	7	7.3

Sources: *WHO (7); **WHO (8); ***UNDP (3); ****WHO (9).

The current health expenditure per capita in Zambia was US$57 in 2016 (9). It consisted of domestic general government health expenditure per capita of US$22; domestic private health expenditure per capita of US$11 (of which US$7 was from out-of-pocket spending); and external health expenditure per capita of US$24. The Zambia current health expenditure per capita was below the range of US$ 76 (minimum) and US$ 342 (maximum) per person per year of health systems investment recommended for attaining health sustainable development goal (SDG) 3 among lower-middle-income countries (10). As a result of underinvestment in national health system, the country has a universal coverage index of 56%, implying a gap in essential health services coverage of 44%.

Second, the inefficiently performing systems that address the social determinants. In 2016, the multidimensional poverty index for Zambia was 0.262; and about 8.86 million people lived in multidimensional poverty (3). As shown in Table 1, less than 50% of population use safely managed drinking-water and sanitation services; 17% of people aged 15 years and above are illiterate; 84% of the population primarily rely on unclean fuels for cooking and heating; 40% of children under five years are stunted due to undernutrition; and 48% of the population feel unsafe.

Third, the underperforming national health research system (NHRS). The goals of a NHRS are to produce health-related evidence and to promote its uptake in health system policy, planning and decision-making (11). In 2014, the Zambia NHRS had a barometer score of 65%, implying it had a performance deficit of 35% (12). Another study conducted in 2018 found Zambia's NHRS barometer score to be 86%, i.e., a 21 percentage point improvement (13).

There is need for increased investments into the national health system, other systems that tackle social determinants of health and NHRS. Currently, the allocation for health system is below the 15% of national budget recommended by the African Heads of State in 2001 (14); and also the recommendation of the Commission on Health Research for Development in 1990 for developing countries to invest at least 2% of national health expenditures in NHRS has not been met (15). The health sector policy-makers ought to use economic evidence-informed messages when advocating with the private sector Chief Executive Officers, ministry of finance, and other relevant sectors ministries for increased investments into health development (16). This is because the latter are not public health specialists, and thus, may not understand public health indices, such as, the DALY.

Some regions, sub-regional economic communities and countries have used evidence on cost-of-illness (direct and indirect costs) when couching their resource mobilization advocacy messages and also to raise public health awareness. In the American region, examples of such studies include total economic costs of illness in 1980 by age and sex (17); economic burden of psoriasis (18); societal cost of heroin use disorder (19); costs of acute hand and wrist injuries (20); economic costs of diabetes (21); economic burden of schizophrenia (22); and economic cost of obesity (23).

Similar studies have been carried out in Europe, for example, on the cost of depression (24); cost of epilepsy (25); cost of disorders of the brain (26); costs of multiple sclerosis (27); economic impact of blindness (28); cost-of-illness of melanoma (29); cost-of-illness in nine Central and Eastern European countries (30); and economic burden of moderate to severe irritable bowel syndrome with constipation (31).

In Africa, a few studies estimated the indirect cost of child mortality (32); Ebola virus disease deaths in West Africa (33); tuberculosis deaths (34); maternal deaths (35); NCD deaths (36); and neglected tropical diseases deaths (37). The main shortcoming of these studies was that they focussed only on economic losses associated with potential years of life lost due to premature mortality, and ignored the years of life lived with non-fatal disability. One regional study estimated the aggregated indirect cost of DALYs lost (38). A few sub-regional studies estimated the monetary value of DALYs lost in 2015, e.g., the East African Community (39); the Arab Maghreb Union (40); and the Economic and Monetary Community of Central Africa (41).

Whereas, the regional and sub-regional aggregated economic studies are useful for advocacy and comparison purposes at those levels, Zambia requires contextualized evidence for national advocacy. To the best of our knowledge, disaggregated evidence on money value of DALYs lost among all age groups and from a wide range of diseases and injuries in Zambia does not exist. Also there is no evidence of the potential money savings assuming the country achieved disease and injury-related SDG3 targets by 2030. Therefore, the aim of the current study was to contribute to bridging these knowledge / information gaps.

The study reported in this paper had three specific objectives. Firstly, to estimate the money value of DALYs lost in Zambia in 2017, using 2019 prices. Second, to estimate the monetary value of DALYs lost in Zambia in 2030, assuming all disease and injury-related SDG3 targets are achieved. Finally, to calculate the potential money savings from DALY losses averted.

OUR STUDY

The World Bank pioneered in 1990 measurement of burden of disease in selected demographic regions using the DALY index (42). Murray (43) provides technical foundation for DALYs. He explains that the DALY captures both premature death and non-fatal health consequences of disease and injury. Thus, DALY is the sum of potential years of life lost (PYLL) due to premature mortality and years of life lived with a disability (YLD).

The study reported in this paper calculates the money value of DALYs lost in Zambia in 2017 from 163 diseases and injuries. The data on number of DALYs lost were extracted from the Institute for Health Metrics and Evaluation (IHME) global burden of disease study 2017 database (4). GBD 2017 DALYs and HALE Collaborators (44) provides details of the methods and sources of data for the Global Burden of Disease Study 2017.

Estimating the money value of the stock DALYs lost in Zambia in 2017

We are interested in estimating the money value of the stock of DALYs lost to Zambian society in 2017. The net output approach first proposed by Weisbrod (45), and subsequently, adapted to monetarily value DALYs in the East African Community (39), the Arab Maghreb Union (40), the Central African Economic and Monetary Community (41), and the African region (38) was applied in this study.

The money value of DALYs lost in Zambia from 163 diseases and injuries (ZEVDALY) is the sum of the money value of DALY losses from each jth disease or injury ($EVDALY_j$). In algebraic terms:

$$ZEVDALY_{2017} = \sum_{i=1}^{k=163}(EVDALY_1 + EVDALY_2 + EVDALY_3 + \cdots + EVDALY_k) \quad (1)$$

where: $\sum_{j=1}^{k=163}$ is the summation of money values of DALYs lost from the first to the one-hundred-sixty-third disease and injury; $EVDALY_1$ is the money value of DALYs from the first disease; $EVDALY_2$ is the money value of DALYs from the second disease; $EVDALY_3$ is the money value of DALYs from the third disease; and $EVDALY_k$ is the money value of DALYs from the kth disease.

The money value of DALYs lost from each of the 163 diseases and injuries is equal to Zambia's per capita GDP (PCGDP) minus current health expenditure per person (CHE) multiplied by the number of DALYs lost from each disease or injury ($DALY_j$). This can be formally expressed as:

$$EVDALY_1 = \{(PCGDP - CHE) \times DALY_1\} \quad (2)$$

$$EVDALY_2 = \{(PCGDP - CHE) \times DALY_2\} \quad (3)$$

$$EVDALY_3 = \{(PCGDP - CHE) \times DALY_3\} \quad (4)$$

$$EVDALY_k = \{(PCGDP - CHE) \times DALY_k\} \quad (5)$$

where: $DALY_1$ is the number of DALYs lost from disease 1, $DALY_2$ is the number of DALYs lost from disease 2, $DALY_3$ is the number of DALYs lost from disease 3, and $DALY_k$ is the number of DALYs lost from k^{th} disease or injury. The DALYs extracted from IHME database were already discounted at 3%.

Algorithm used in estimating expected money value of DALY losses in 2030

This subsection presents formulas used in estimating the money value DALY losses in 2030 assuming the five disease-related SDG3 targets in Box 1 are fully achieved in Zambia.

We estimated using equations 6 to 13 the expected 2030 money values of DALYs lost, assuming the SDG targets for maternal mortality ratio (Target 3.1); neonatal mortality (Target 3.2); and HIV/AIDS, tuberculosis, malaria, neglected tropical diseases (NTDs) and viral hepatitis deaths (target 3.3) will be fully achieved.

Box 1. Health SDG3 targets and expected percentage reductions for Zambia

Target	Description	Percentage reduction envisaged in SDG targets
SDG 3.1	By 2030, reduce the global maternal mortality ratio to less than 70 per 100,000 live births (7, 46). Average Annual Rate of Reduction (AARR) formula (47).	68.75% (AARR= 7.972450318%)
SDG 3.2	By 2030, end preventable deaths of newborns, with all countries aiming to reduce neonatal mortality to at least as low as 12 per 1,000 live births (7, 46).	45.45% (AARR=4.237154909%)
SDG 3.3	By 2030, end the epidemics of AIDS, tuberculosis, malaria and neglected tropical diseases and reduce hepatitis, water-borne diseases and other communicable diseases (46).	
	(a). Reduce global HIV-related deaths from 1,062,352 in 2015 to below 500,000 by 2020 (48).	54.55% (AARR=5.476185967%)
	(b). Malaria mortality rates will be reduced globally by at least 90% from 2015 to 2030 (49, 50).	90% (AARR=15.17%)
	(c). The number of tuberculosis (TB) deaths will be reduced by 90% from 2015 to 2030 (51, 52).	90% (AARR=15.17%)
	(d). Mortality due to vector-borne diseases will be reduced globally by at least 75% from 2016 to 2030 (4, 53).	75% (AARR=9.427633574%)
	(e). Globally reduce viral hepatitis B and C deaths from 1.4 million deaths reduced to less than 500,000 by 2030 (54).	64.29% (AARR=7.090496208%)
SDG 3.4	By 2030, reduce premature mortality due to NCDs by one third through prevention and treatment and promote mental health and well-being (4, 46).	33.3% (AARR=2.854607339%)
SDG 3.6	By 2020, halve the number of global deaths and injuries from road traffic accidents (4, 7, 46).	50% (AARR=4.830484699%

SDG 3 target 3.1: reduce the money value of DALYs from maternal disorders

$$EVDALY_{MD2030} = EVDALY_{MD2017} - \left[EVDALY_{MD2017} \times \left(\frac{MM_{2017} - MM_{T3.1}}{MM_{2017}}\right)\right] \quad (6)$$

where: $EVDALY_{MD2030}$ is the expected money value of DALYs lost from maternal disorders in 2030; $EVDALY_{MD2017}$ is the money value of DALYs lost from maternal disorders in 2017; MM_{2017} is the maternal mortality ratio in 2017; T3.1 is the SDG3 target 3.1 on maternal mortality ratio; and $MM_{T3.1}$ is expected maternal mortality ratio in 2030 supposing target 3.1 is achieved. For instance:

$$MVDALY_{MD2030} = Int\$919{,}956{,}631 - \left[Int\$919{,}956{,}631 \times \left(\frac{510-70}{510}\right)\right] = Int\$126{,}268{,}557.$$

SDG 3 target 3.2: reduce the money value of DALYs from neonatal disorders

$$EVDALY_{ND2030} = EVDALY_{ND2017} - \left[EVDALY_{ND2017} \times \left(\frac{NN_{2017} - NN_{T3.2}}{NN_{2017}}\right)\right] \quad (7)$$

where: $EVDALY_{ND2030}$ is the expected money value of DALYs lost from neonatal disorders in 2030; $EVDALY_{ND2017}$ is the money value of DALYs lost from neonatal disorders in 2017; NN_{2017} is the neonatal mortality ratio in 2017; T3.2 is the SDG3 target 3.2 on neonatal mortality rate; and $NN_{T3.2}$ is the expected neonatal mortality rate in 2030 assuming target 3.2 is achieved.

SDG 3 target 3.3a: reduce the money value of DALYs from HIV

$$EVDALY_{HIV2030} = EVDALY_{HIV2017} - \left[EVDALY_{HIV2017} \times \left(\frac{HIVD_{2017} - HIVD_{T3.3a}}{HIVD_{2017}}\right)\right] \quad (8)$$

where: $EVDALY_{HIV2030}$ is the expected money value of DALYs lost from HIV/AIDS in 2030; $EVDALY_{HIV2017}$ is the money value of DALYs lost from HIV/AIDS in 2017; $HIVD_{2017}$ is the number of HIV/AIDS deaths in 2017; T3.3a is the SDG3 target 3.3a on HIV deaths; and $HIVD_{T3.2}$ is the expected number of HIV/AIDS deaths in 2030 if target 3.3a is achieved.

SDG 3 target 3.3b: reduce the money value of DALYs from malaria

$$EVDALY_{MAL2030} = EVDALY_{MAL2017} - \left[EVDALY_{MAL2017} \times \left(\frac{DMA_{2017} - DMA_{T3.3b}}{DMA_{2017}}\right)\right] \quad (9)$$

where: $EVDALY_{MAL2030}$ is the expected money value of DALYs lost from malaria in 2030; $EVDALY_{MAL2017}$ is the money value of DALYs lost from malaria in 2017; DMA_{2017} is the number of deaths from malaria in 2017; T3.3b is the SDG3 target 3.3b on malaria deaths; and $DMA_{T3.3b}$ is the number of deaths from malaria in 2030 if target 3.3b is achieved.

SDG 3 target 3.3c: reduce the money value of DALYs from tuberculosis (TB)

$$EVDALY_{TB2030} = EVDALY_{TB2017} - \left[EVDALY_{TB2017} \times \left(\frac{DTB_{2017} - DTB_{T3.3C}}{DTB_{2017}}\right)\right] \quad (10)$$

where: $EVDALY_{TB2030}$ is the expected money value of DALYs lost from TB in 2030; $EVDALY_{TBD2017}$ is the money value of DALYs lost from TB in 2017; DTB_{2017} is the number of deaths from TB in 2017; T3.3c is the SDG3 target 3.3c on TB deaths; and $DTB_{T3.3c}$ is the number of deaths from TB in 2030, if target 3.3c is reached.

SDG 3 target 3.3d: reduce the money value of DALYs from neglected tropical disease (NTD)

$$EVDALY_{NTDD2030} = EVDALY_{NTDD2017} - \left[EVDALY_{NTDD2017} \times \left(\frac{DNT_{2017} - DNT_{T3.3d}}{DNT_{2017}}\right)\right] \tag{11}$$

where: $EVDALY_{NTDD2030}$ is the expected money value of DALYs lost from NTD in 2030; $EVDALY_{NTDD2017}$ is the money value of DALYs lost from NTD in 2017; DNT_{2017} is the number of deaths from NTD in 2017; T3.3d is the SDG3 target 3.3d on NTD deaths; and $DNT_{T3.3d}$ is the expected number of deaths from NTD in 2030, assuming target 3.3d is realized.

SDG 3 target 3.3e: reduce the money value of DALYs from viral hepatitis (VH)

$$EVDALY_{VH2030} = EVDALY_{VH2017} - \left[EVDALY_{VH2017} \times \left(\frac{DVH_{2017} - DVH_{T3.3e}}{DVH_{2017}}\right)\right] \tag{12}$$

where: $EVDALY_{VH2030}$ is the expected money value of DALYs lost from viral hepatitis (VH) in 2030; $EVDALY_{VH2017}$ is the money value of DALYs lost from VH in 2017; DVH_{2017} is the number of deaths from VH in 2017; T3.3e is the SDG3 target 3.3e on VH deaths; and $DVH_{T3.3e}$ is the expected number of deaths from VH in 2030, if target 3.3e is accomplished.

SDG 3 target 3.4: reduce the money value of DALYs from NCD

$$EVDALY_{NCD2030} = EVDALY_{NCD2017} - \left[EVDALY_{NCD2017} \times \left(\frac{DNC_{2017} - DNC_{T3.4}}{DNC_{2017}}\right)\right] \quad (13)$$

where: $EVDALY_{NCD2030}$ is the expected money value of DALYs lost from NCD in 2030; $EVDALY_{NCD2017}$ is the money value of DALYs lost from NCD in 2017; DNC_{2017} is the number of deaths from NCD in 2017; T3.4 is the SDG3 target 3.4 on NCD deaths; and $NCD_{T3.4}$ is the number of deaths from NCD in 2030, assuming target 3.4 is achieved.

SDG 3 target 3.6: reduce the money value of DALYs from transport injury

$$EVDALY_{TID2030} = EVDALY_{TID2017} - \left[EVDALY_{TID2017} \times \left(\frac{DTI_{2017} - DTI_{T3.6}}{DTI_{2017}}\right)\right] \quad (14)$$

where: $EVDALY_{TID2030}$ is the expected money value of DALYs from transport injuries in 2030; $EVDALY_{TID2017}$ is the money value of DALYs from transport injuries in 2017; DTI_{2017} is the number of deaths from transport injuries in 2017; T3.6 is the SDG3 target 3.6 on transport injury deaths; and $DTI_{T3.6}$ is the number of deaths from transport injuries in 2030, assuming target 3.6 is achieved.

Calculate the potential money savings from DALY losses averted

The expected savings in money value of DALYs loss averted assuming full achievement of jth SDG3 disease (or injury) target was estimated by subtracting the money value of DALYs lost in 2017 from the money value of DALYs lost in 2030 from j^{th} disease (or injury).

For example, the expected savings in money value of DALYs lost from HIV/AIDS was calculated as follows:

$$EVDALY_{HIV-SAVINGS} = (EVDALY_{HIV2017} - EVDALY_{HIV2030}) \quad (15)$$

$$EVDALY_{HIV-SAVINGS} = (\text{Int\$}5{,}963{,}300{,}037 - Int\$2{,}710{,}590{,}926) = Int\$3{,}252{,}709{,}111\,.$$

where: $EVDALY_{HIV\text{-}SAVINGS}$ are the expected savings the money value of DALYs loss from HIV/AIDS premature deaths and disability averted; $EVDALY_{HIV2030}$ is the money value of DALYs expected to be lost from HIV/AIDS premature deaths and disability in 2030; and $EVDALY_{HIV2017}$ is the money value of DALYs lost from HIV/AIDS premature deaths and disability in 2017.

Data sources and software

The Int$4,264 per capita GDP data was extracted from the International Monetary Fund world world outlook database (2); the Int$175 current health expenditure per capita data was gotten from the WHO Global Health Expenditure Database (9); and the DALY data for the 163 diseases and injuries was obtained from the IHME Global Burden of Disease Study 2017 database (4). The money model containing the aforementioned 14 equations was estimated using the Excel Software developed by Microsoft (New York).

FINDINGS

In 2017, the country lost a total of 7,919,620 DALYs from all causes with a money value of Int$32,385,080,324.

Of which, Int$20,248,590,452 (62.5%) was attributed to CMNN; Int$10,109,674,684 (31.2%) to NCD; and Int$ 2,026,815,188 (6.3%) to INJ.

Communicable, maternal, neonatal and nutritional diseases

Out of the Int$20.25 billion from CMNN, 31.2% resulted from HIV/AIDS and sexually transmitted infections; 18.6% from respiratory infections and tuberculosis; 11.16% from enteric infections; 7.9% from neglected tropical diseases and malaria; 5.1% from other infectious diseases; 19.3% from maternal and neonatal disorders; and 6.6% from nutritional deficiencies. Figure 1 shows the money value of DALYs lost from CMNN. Malaria, tuberculosis, diarrheal diseases, lower respiratory infections, neonatal disorders and HIV/AIDS alone account for 83% of the CMNN money value of DALYs lost.

HIV/AIDS and sexually transmitted infections

The money value of DALYs lost from HIV/AIDS and sexually transmitted infections was Int$6,320,634,532. HIV/AIDS and sexually transmitted infections (excluding HIV) accounted for 94.3% and 5.7%, respectively.

Respiratory infections and tuberculosis

The respiratory infections and tuberculosis caused DALYs loss worth Int$ 3,765,542,738. Of which, 58.3% emanated from lower respiratory infections, 38.7% from tuberculosis, 2.4% from upper respiratory infections, and 0.6% from otitis media.

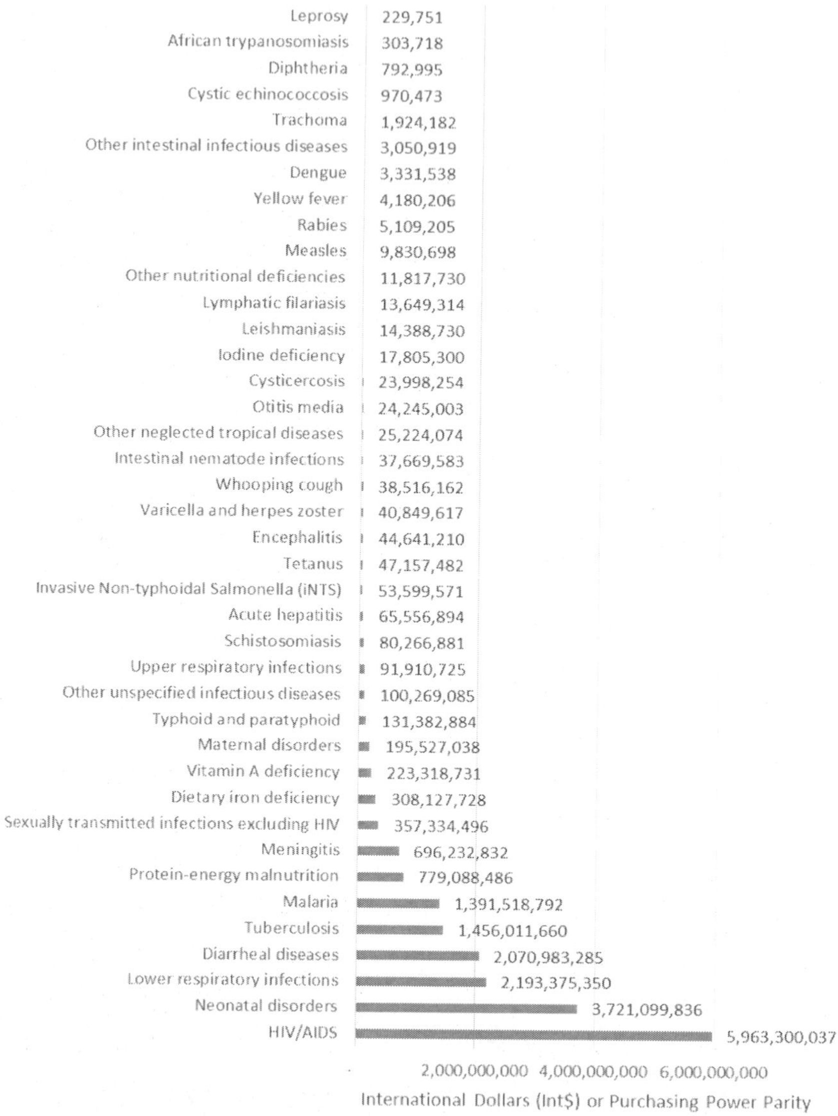

Source: Authors estimates.

Figure 1. Money value of DALYs lost from communicable, maternal, neonatal and nutritional diseases (2019 Int$ or PPP).

Enteric infections

The enteric infections bled DALYs with a value of Int$ 2,259,016,659. Out of that, 91.7% was from diarrheal diseases, 5.8% from typhoid and paratyphoid, 2.4% invasive non-typhoidal salmonella (iNTS), and 0.1% from other intestinal infectious diseases.

Neglected tropical diseases (NTD) and malaria

The NTDs and malaria inflicted DALY losses valued at Int$1,602,764,699. Malaria alone accounted for DALYs worth Int$ 1,391,518,792 (86.8%); and NTDs led to DALY loss valued at Int$211,245,907 (13.2%). Table 2 shows the distribution of money values across the different NTDs. Schistosomiasis, intestinal nematode infections and cysticercosis alone accounted for 67.2% of the money value of DALYs lost from NTDs.

Table 2. Money value of DALYs lost from NTDs (Int$, 2019)

Diseases	Money value in Int$	Percent
Schistosomiasis	80,266,881	38.0
Intestinal nematode infections	37,669,583	17.8
Cysticercosis	23,998,254	11.4
Leishmaniasis	14,388,730	6.8
Lymphatic filariasis	13,649,314	6.5
Rabies	5,109,205	2.4
Yellow fever	4,180,206	2.0
Dengue	3,331,538	1.6
Trachoma	1,924,182	0.9
Cystic echinococcosis	970,473	0.5
African trypanosomiasis	303,718	0.1
Leprosy	229,751	0.1
Other neglected tropical diseases	25,224,074	11.9
TOTAL	211,245,907	100.0

Source: Authors estimates.

Other infectious diseases

As shown in Table 3, the other infectious diseases haemorrhaged DALYs with a value of Int$ 1,043,846,975. Meningitis and acute hepatitis alone accounted for 73%.

Table 3. Money value of DALYs lost from other infectious diseases (Int$, 2019)

Disease	Money value in Int$	Percent
Meningitis	696,232,832	66.7
Other unspecified infectious diseases	100,269,085	9.6
Acute hepatitis	65,556,894	6.3
Tetanus	47,157,482	4.5
Encephalitis	44,641,210	4.3
Varicella and herpes zoster	40,849,617	3.9
Whooping cough	38,516,162	3.7
Measles	9,830,698	0.9
Diphtheria	792,995	0.1
TOTAL	1,043,846,975	100

Source: Authors estimates.

Maternal and neonatal disorders: The maternal and neonatal disorders caused a loss in DALYs valued at Int$ 3,916,626,874. Out of which, 95% and 5% of the money value of DALY lost was attributed to neonatal disorders and maternal disorders, respectively.

Nutritional deficiencies: The nutritional deficiencies resulted in DALY losses valued at Int$1,340,157,975. Out of which, 58.1% was attributed to DALYs lost from protein-energy malnutrition, 23% from dietary iron deficiency, 16.7% from vitamin A deficiency, 1.3% from iodine deficiency, and 0.9% from other nutritional deficiencies.

Non-communicable diseases

Of the Int$10.11 billion (31.2%) NCDs, 12.6% was attributed to neoplasms; 13.3% to cardiovascular diseases; 4.7% to chronic respiratory diseases; 8.5% to digestive diseases; 8.9% to neurological disorders; 9.1% to mental disorders; 2.3% to substance use disorders; 7.1% to diabetes and kidney diseases; 4.6% to diabetes and kidney diseases; 3.2% to sense organ diseases; 5.4% to musculoskeletal disorders; and 20.2% to other NCDs.

Neoplasms

Figure 2 shows the money value of DALYs lost from neoplasms was Int$ 1,278,378,790. About 40.8% of that money value was from liver cancer, leukaemia, breast cancer, non-Hodgkin lymphoma and cervical cancer.

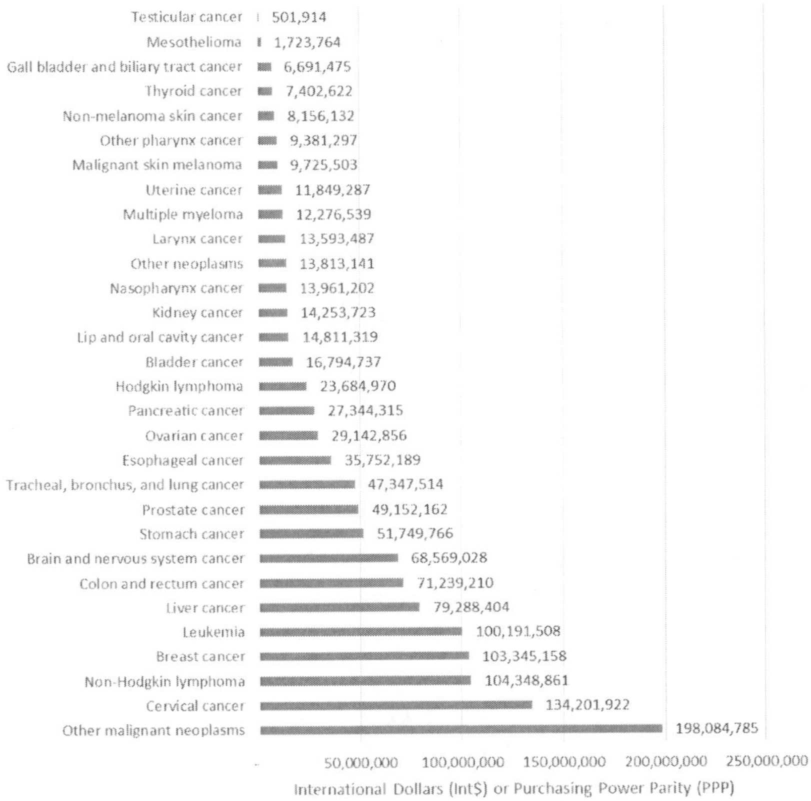

Source: Authors estimates.

Figure 2. Money value of DALYs lost from neoplasms (2019 Int$ or PPP).

Cardiovascular diseases

Figure 3 shows the money value of DALYs lost from cardiovascular diseases was Int$ 1,348,383,417. Approximately, 81.5% of that money value was from hypertensive heart disease, stroke and ischemic heart disease.

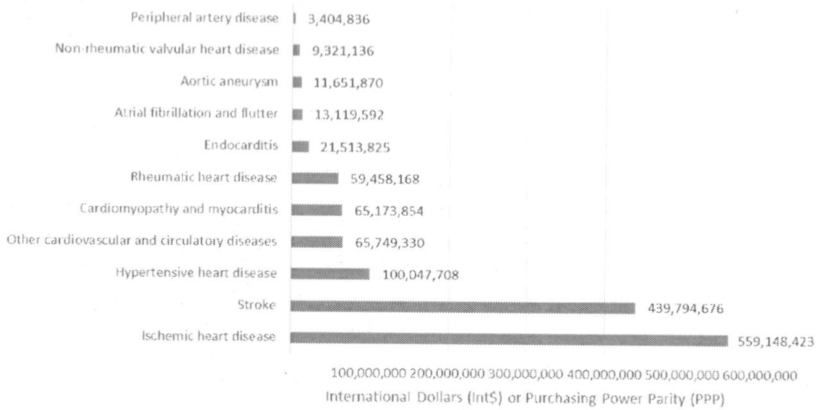

Source: Authors estimates.

Figure 3. Money value of DALYs lost from cardiovascular diseases (2019 Int$ or PPP).

Chronic respiratory diseases

The money value of DALYs lost from chronic respiratory diseases was Int$478,995,712. Almost 46.4% of that money value was from chronic obstructive pulmonary disease; 45.4% from asthma; 1.6% from interstitial lung disease and pulmonary sarcoidosis; 0.4% from pneumoconiosis; and 6.2% from other chronic respiratory diseases.

Digestive diseases

Figure 4 depicts the money value of DALYs lost from digestive diseases was Int$860,413,297. Upper digestive system diseases and cirrhosis plus other chronic liver diseases account for 72.9% of the money value of DALYs lost from digestive diseases.

Neurological disorders

The money value of DALYs lost from neurological disorders was Int$898,608,941. Nearly, 47.0% of that money value was from headache disorders; 35.0% from epilepsy; 8.9% from Alzheimer's disease and other dementias; 1.6% from Parkinson's disease; 0.3% from multiple sclerosis; 0.04% from motor neuron disease; and 7.2% from other neurological disorders.

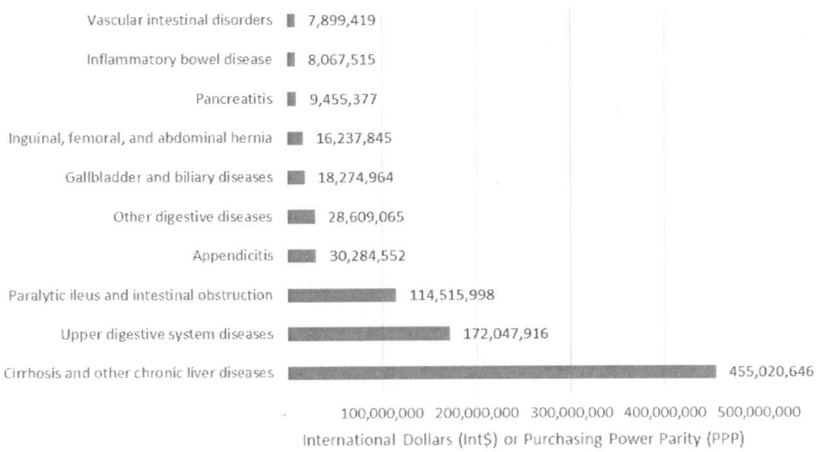

Source: Authors estimates.

Figure 4. Money value of DALYs lost from digestive diseases (2019 Int$ or PPP).

Mental disorders

Figure 5 shows the money value of DALYs lost from mental disorders was Int$ 917,761,126. The depressive disorders, anxiety disorders and conduct disorder accounted for 67.5% of that money value.

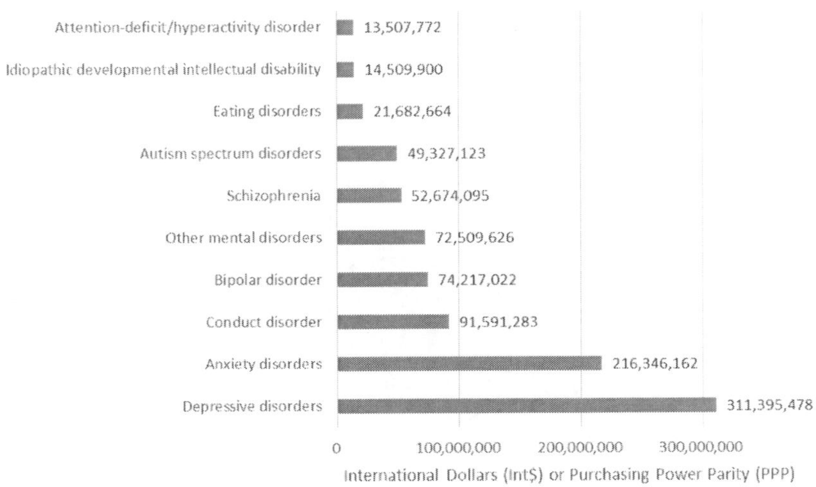

Source: Authors estimates.

Figure 5. Money value of DALYs lost from mental disorders (2019 Int$ or PPP).

Substance use disorders

The money value of DALYs lost from substance use disorders was Int$230,933,197. Alcohol use disorders and drug use disorders accounted for 53% and 47%, respectively.

Diabetes and kidney diseases

The money value of DALYs lost from diabetes and kidney diseases was Int$713,914,222. Out of that money value, diabetes mellitus accounted for 60.5%, chronic kidney disease for 39.1% and acute glomerulonephritis for 0.4%.

Skin and subcutaneous diseases

Figure 6 portrays the money value of DALYs lost from skin and subcutaneous diseases was Int$ 468,317,124. Dermatitis, urticaria, fungal skin diseases, and viral skin diseases made up 66.2% of the money value.

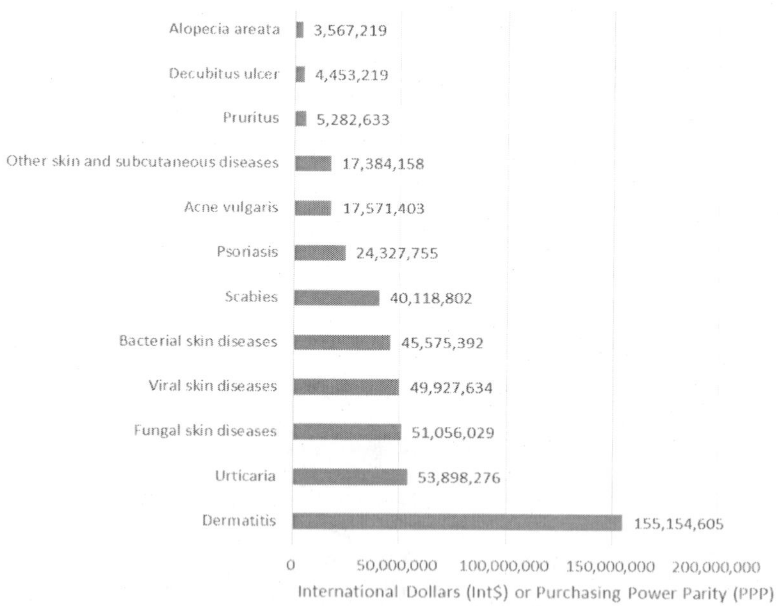

Source: Authors estimates.

Figure 6. Money value of DALYs lost from skin and subcutaneous diseases (2019 Int$ or PPP).

Sense organ diseases

The money value of DALYs lost from sense organ diseases was Int$323,481,482. Out of that money value, 39.3% was attributed to blindness and vision impairment; 56.7% to age-related and other hearing loss; and 4% to other sense organ diseases.

Musculoskeletal disorders

The money value of DALYs lost from Musculoskeletal disorders was Int$546,699,206. Approximately, 59.7% of the money value was attributed to low back pain, 18% to neck pain, 4.1% to osteoarthritis, 3.1% to rheumatoid arthritis, 0.8% to gout, and 14.3% to other musculoskeletal disorders.

Other non-communicable diseases

The money value of DALYs lost from other NCDs was Int$2,043,788,169. Out of that money value, 75.9% was due to congenital birth defects; 5.7% to urinary diseases and male infertility; 4.8% to haemoglobinopathies and haemolytic anaemias; 3.8% to gynaecological diseases; 3.8% to oral disorders; 2.3% to endocrine, metabolic, blood, and immune disorders; and 3.7% to sudden infant death syndrome.

Injuries

Of the money value of Int$ 2.03 billion from injuries, 27.8% was attributed to transport injuries, 47.7% from unintentional injuries and 24.5% from self-harm and interpersonal violence. Figure 7 indicates the money value of DALYs lost from various forms of injuries.

Unintentional injuries

The money value of DALYs lost from unintentional injuries was Int$ 966,626,418. Out of which, 22.7% was attributed to falls; 18.8% to drowning; 15.7% to fire, heat, and hot substances; 12.4% to exposure to mechanical forces; 6.5% to adverse effects of medical treatment; 6% to animal contact; 5.6% foreign body; 5.1% poisonings; 1.6% to environmental heat and cold exposure; 0.01% to exposure to forces of nature; and 5.59% to other unintentional injuries. Therefore, 53.9% of that was ascribed to falls, drowning, and exposure to mechanical forces alone.

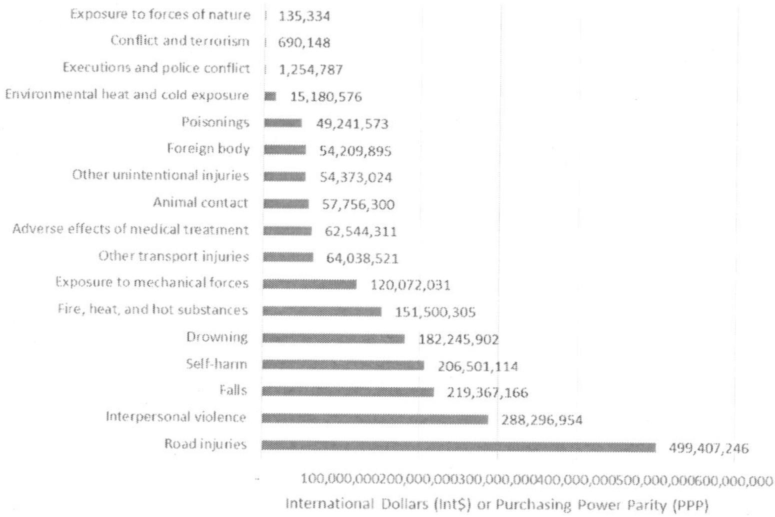

Source: Authors estimates.

Figure 7. Money value of DALYs lost from various forms of injuries (2019 Int$ or PPP).

Transport injuries

The money value of DALYs lost from transport injuries was Int$563,445,767. Of this, 88.6% was attributed to road injuries and 11.4% to other transport injuries.

Self-harm and interpersonal violence

Self-harm and interpersonal injuries resulted in a DALY loss valued at Int$496,743,002. Out of which, 58% was due to interpersonal violence, 41.6% to self-harm, 0.3% to executions and police conflict, and 0.1% to conflict and terrorism.

Expected money value of DALY losses in 2030

Table 4 shows the money value of DALYs lost in 2017, money value of DALYs lost in 2030, and expected savings from DALYs averted assuming the five SDG3 targets are achieved.

Table 4. Money value of DALYs lost distributed by SDG health conditions

Health condition/diseases	(A). Money Value of DALYS lost in 2017 (Int$)	(B). Money Value of DALYS lost in 2030 (Int$)	(C). Reduction/Savings in Money Value of DALYS lost in 2030 (Int$) [C=A-B)]
SDG 3.1: Maternal disorders	195,527,038	61,102,199	134,424,839
SDG 3.2: Neonatal disorders	3,721,099,836	2,029,690,820	1,691,409,016
SDG 3.3: Tuberculosis	1,456,011,660	145,601,166	1,310,410,494
SDG 3.3: HIV/AIDS	5,963,300,037	2,710,590,925.71	3,252,709,111
SDG 3.3: Malaria	1,391,518,792	139,151,879	1,252,366,913
SDG 3.3: Acute hepatitis	65,556,894	23,413,176	42,143,717
SDG 3.3: NTDs (a+b..+l)	211,245,907	52,811,477	158,434,430
(a). Schistosomiasis	80,266,881	20,066,720	60,200,161
(b). Intestinal nematode infections	37,669,583	9,417,396	28,252,187
(c). Cysticercosis	23,998,254	5,999,564	17,998,691
(d). Leishmaniasis	14,388,730	3,597,182	10,791,547
(e). Lymphatic filariasis	13,649,314	3,412,328	10,236,985
(f). Rabies	5,109,205	1,277,301	3,831,903
(g). Yellow fever	4,180,206	1,045,051	3,135,154
(h). Dengue	3,331,538	832,884	2,498,653
(i). Trachoma	1,924,182	481,046	1,443,137
(j). Cystic echinococcosis	970,473	242,618	727,855
(k). African trypanosomiasis	303,718	75,930	227,789
(l). Leprosy	229,751	57,438	172,313
(m). Other neglected tropical diseases	25,224,074	6,306,018	18,918,055
SDG 3.4: Non-communicable diseases (a+b+c+..+l)	10,109,674,684	6,739,816,822	3,369,857,863
(a). Neoplasms	1,278,378,790.4	852,256,788	426,122,002
(b). Cardiovascular Diseases	1,348,383,417.4	898,926,773	449,456,645
(c) Chronic respiratory diseases	478,995,712.3	319,332,072	159,663,641
(d). Digestive diseases	860,413,297.4	573,611,733	286,801,564

Table 4. (Continued)

Health condition/diseases	(A). Money Value of DALYS lost in 2017 (Int$)	(B). Money Value of DALYS lost in 2030 (Int$)	(C). Reduction/Savings in Money Value of DALYS lost in 2030 (Int$) [C=A-B)]
(e).Neurological Disorders	898,608,940.7	599,075,622	299,533,318
(f). Mental Disorders	917,761,125.6	611,843,810	305,917,316
(g). Substance Use Disorders	230,933,197.4	153,956,235	76,976,963
(h). Diabetes and Kidney Diseases	713,914,221.6	475,945,194	237,969,027
(i). Skin and Subcutaneous Diseases	468,317,124.4	312,212,977	156,104,147
(j). Sense Organ Diseases	323,481,482.5	215,655,400	107,826,083
(k). Musculoskeletal Disorders	546,699,205.9	364,467,960	182,231,246
(l).Other non-communicable diseases	2,043,788,168.8	1,362,532,258	681,255,910
SDG 3.6: Transport injuries	563,445,767	281,722,884	281,722,884
TOTAL (INT$)	25,140,750,036	12,183,901,349	12,956,848,687

Source: Authors estimates.

Discussion

In 2017, the country lost a total of 7,919,620 DALYs from all causes with a total money value of Int$32,385,080,324. Of the latter, 62.5% resulted from CMNN, 31.2% from NCDs and 6.3% from INJ. About 12,853,546,433 (39.7%) of the money value of DALYs lost was sustained among the 15-59 years old, i.e., the most economically productive age bracket.

Approximately, Int$25.14 billion (77.63%) of the total money value of DALYs lost in Zambia was related to SDG 3 targets 3.1, 3.2, 3.3, 3.4 and 3.6 diseases and injuries. Our study revealed that, full achievement of the five SDG 3 targets would lead to an estimated Int$ 13 billion (51.54%) decrease in the money value of SDG3-related DALYs lost by 2030.

SDG 3.1 and SDG 3.2: Maternal and neonatal disorders

Full achievement of SDG3 targets 3.1 and 3.2 by 2030 would annually avert DALY loss with a money value of Int$1.826 billion. The expected saving might be achieved if the reproductive, maternal, child, and adolescent health and nutrition services planned for in chapter 4 of the Zambia national health strategic plan 2017-2021 (5); the comprehensive immunization multi-year plan 2011-2015 (55); the reproductive, maternal, new-born, child and adolescent health and nutrition communication and advocacy strategy 2018-2021 (56); the national maternal and neonatal services referral guidelines (57); the adolescent health strategic plan 2011 to 2015 (58); the new-born health care framework (59); and the national food and nutrition strategic plan for Zambia 2011-2015 (60) are fully implemented in all the 10 provinces in Zambia.

There exists legal framework that undergird implementation of those policy and strategic documents, including the national health services Act (61); the medical and allied professions Act (62); the nurses and midwives Bill (63); and the protection of traditional knowledge, genetic resources and expressions of folklore Act (64).

The Zambia maternal, new-born, child and adolescent health (MNCAH) policies and strategies plans are consistent with pertinent Assembly of African Union (AU) decisions and declarations, e.g., the Maputo plan of action for the operationalisation of the continental policy framework for sexual and reproductive health and rights 2007-2010 (65); the decision on the Report of the Implementation Status of Decision Assembly/AU/Dec.204 (XI) on promotion of maternal, infant and child health and development in Africa (66); the Campaign for Accelerated Reduction of Maternal Mortality (CARMA) (67); the actions on maternal, new-born and child health and development in Africa by 2015 (68); the decision on the reduction of maternal, new-born and child mortality and morbidity in Africa (69); Declaration on Ending Preventable Child and Maternal Death in Africa (70); the decision on progress on maternal, new born and child health (71); the decision on galvanizing political commitment towards the elimination of female genital mutilation in Africa

(72); and the declaration on addressing social determinants of health in Africa - adoption of health in all policies approach (73).

In addition, the Zambia MNCAH policies and strategies plans were informed by relevant resolutions of the United Nations General Assembly (UNGA), including the ones on preventable maternal mortality and morbidity and human rights (74, 75); report of the Office of the United Nations High Commissioner for Human Rights on preventable maternal mortality and morbidity and human rights (76); elimination of preventable maternal mortality and morbidity and the empowerment of women (77); intensification of efforts to end obstetric fistula (78); intensification of efforts to prevent and eliminate all forms of violence against women and girls - domestic violence (79); the rights of the child (80); the child, early and forced marriage (81); intensifying global efforts for the elimination of female genital mutilation (82); and intensification of efforts to prevent and eliminate all forms of violence against women and girls - sexual harassment (83).

The Zambia MNCAH plans are also buttressed by World Health Assembly (WHA) resolutions on reduction of perinatal and neonatal mortality (84); infant and young child nutrition (85, 86, 87), immunization (88, 89) and medicines for children (90); global strategy for women's, children's and adolescents' health (91); global plan of action to strengthen the role of the health system within a national multi-sectoral response to address interpersonal violence, in particular against women and girls, and against children (92); and strengthening integrated, people-centred health services (93).

SDG 3.3: Tuberculosis, HIV/AIDS, malaria, acute hepatitis and NTDs

The attainment of SDG target 3.3 by 2030 would potentially avert DALYs valued at Int$1.31 billion from TB, Int$3.25 billion from HIV/AIDS, Int$1.25 billion from malaria, Int$42.14 million from acute hepatitis and Int$158.43 million from NTDS. Thus, the country may potentially save

DALYs with total money value of Int$6.02 billion. Such a saving might be realized, if communicable disease control services planned for in chapter 4 of the Zambia national health strategic plan 2017-2021 (5); the national HIV/AIDS/STI/TB policy (94); the HIV and AIDS policy for the transport sector (95); the comprehensive HIV prevention roadmap 2017-2021 (96); the national malaria elimination strategic plan 2017–2021 (97); and the Ministry of Health elimination of neglected tropical diseases national masterplan 2019 – 2023 (98). The implementation of communicable diseases strategies and plans is bolstered with pertinent legal framework, including the Public Health Act (99) and the National HIV/AIDS/STI/TB Council Act (100).

The implementation of the abovementioned Zambia policies, strategies and plans for communicable diseases is buttressed with a number of pertinent AU political decisions/declarations, including the Abuja declaration on HIV/AIDS, tuberculosis and other related infections (101); decision on the continental framework for harmonization of approaches among member states, and integration of policies on human rights and people infected and affected by HIV/AIDS in Africa (102); decision on Abuja call for accelerated action towards universal access to HIV/AIDS, tuberculosis and malaria services in Africa (103,104); declaration Assembly/AU/Decl. 2(XIX) on the Report of AIDS Watch Africa Action Committee of Heads of State and Government (105). In addition, Zambia's policies and strategies are also shored up by the WHA resolutions, for example, the global health sector strategies on HIV, viral hepatitis and sexually transmitted infections 2016-2021 (106); the global technical strategy and targets for malaria 2016–2030 (107); and the global vector-borne diseases integrated control response (108).

Furthermore, the Zambia communicable disease control policies and strategies are supported bolstered by the UNGA declarations/resolutions on intensifying efforts to end HIV and AIDS epidemic by 2030 (109); fight against tuberculosis (110); antimicrobial resistance (111); accelerating efforts to control and eliminate malaria (112); and NTDs (113).

SDG 3.4: Non-communicable diseases

Zambia would potentially avert DALYs with a money value of Int$3.37 billion, if the country succeeds to decrease NCDs burden by one third by 2030 (SDG3 target 3.4). Were Zambia to make universally available and accessible health services planned for in the NCD strategic plan 2013-2016 (114); the cancer control strategic plan 2016-2021 (115); the national health strategic plan 2017-2021 (5); and the health in all policies strategic framework 2017-2021 (116), the country might stand a good chance of achieving the SDG3 target 3.4. The implementation of NCD strategies and plans is underpinned by a few laws, such as, the mental health Act (117), the ionising radiation protection Act (118), and the occupational health and safety Act (119).

The Zambian NCD policies and strategies were partly informed by the WHA resolutions on global strategy for the prevention and control of NCD (120); framework convention on tobacco control (121); strategies to reduce the harmful use of alcohol (122); implementation of the global NCD strategy (123); follow-up to the political declaration of the high-level meeting of the UNGA on prevention and control of NCDs (124); global action plan for the prevention and control of NCDs (125); mental health action plan 2013–2020 (126); eye health global action plan (127); health impact of air pollution (128); global strategy and action plan on ageing and health (129); cancer prevention and control (130); global action plan on dementia (131); and the global action plan on physical activity (132).

The UNGA resolutions A/RES/66/2 (133), A/RES/72/274 (134), A/RES/72/144 (135), and A/RES/72/306 (136) commits the Zambian Head of State and Government to provide high-level leadership in the fight against NCDs and in addressing issues related to ageing and nutrition.

SDG 3.6: Transport injuries

Were Zambia to be successful in reducing by half the transport-related injuries, it could potentially avert DALYs with a money value of Int$

281.72 million. In order to reduce the disability and deaths from transport-related injuries, the Government of Zambia developed a national road safety policy, strategy and action plan with six groups of measures, including enhancing road safety management, safer roads and mobility, safer vehicles, safer road users, post-crash response, and improving enforcement (137). The implementation of road safety policy framework is guided and regulated by the Road Traffic Act No. 11 of 2002 (138). Among others, the law stipulates the penalties for careless driving, reckless (or dangerous driving), being in charge of motor vehicle when under influence of drink or drugs, driving when under influence of drink or drugs, and causing death by reckless (or dangerous) driving of motor vehicles (138). The Zambia policy, strategy and plan were informed by the Sixty-ninth WHA resolution on the second global high-level conference on road safety (139).

The Zambia road safety policy framework is reinforced by the UNGA resolution A/RES/64/255 that proclaimed the period 2011–2020 as the Decade of Action for Road Safety (140). The UNGA resolutions A/RES/66/260 (141), A/RES/68/269 (142), A/RES/70/260 (143) and A/RES/72/271 (144) labelled "improving global road safety" provides additional high-level political support for sustained implementation of policy, strategies and action plans for curbing disability and mortality from transport related injuries.

Limitations of the study

Limitations in calculation of DALY

As mentioned earlier, the DALY has two components, the YLD and YLL from premature mortality. According to the GBD 2017 Mortality Collaborators, estimation of the latter component used data from a combination of sources:

> "Data used include vital registration systems, sample registration systems, household surveys (complete birth histories, summary birth

histories, sibling histories), censuses (summary birth histories, household deaths), and Demographic Surveillance Sites (p.1684) (145).

Due to fragility of vital registration systems, completeness of cause-of-death primary data in the WHO African Region is 6%, compared to 49% in the world and 97% in the European Region (7). Therefore, the information on numbers and causes of deaths were obtained using second-best approaches, which affects the veracity of DALY estimates.

The GBD 2017 Mortality Collaborators (145), GBD 2017 DALYs and HALE Collaborators (146) and GBD 2017 Disease and Injury Incidence and Prevalence Collaborators (147) discusses additional limitations surrounding calculations of DALYs in the Global Burden of Disease Study 2017.

Limitations in GDP estimations:

This study used GDP per capita to value the DALYs lost into their money equivalents. The calculations of GDP omit all non-money production, including work done at home, e.g., childcare, caring for the elderly, cooking, fetching water and collecting firewood; overlooks consequences of ecological, socioeconomic and political inequities; and ignores environmental cost of economic production processes (148).

CONCLUSION

Diseases and injuries inflicts a heavy burden on the health and economy of Zambia every year. Full attainment of the SDG3 targets 3.1, 3.2, 3.3, 3.4 and 3.6 would save the country about Int$13 billion, i.e., 16.6% of the total GDP of Zambia in 2019.

There is no shortage of policies and strategies at national, continental and global levels for tackling the burden of disease and injuries. Health-related policies and strategies are not adequately resourced to ensure their full implementation.

Therefore, there is urgent need for the Zambian Government, the domestic private sector and the development partners to increase investments into strengthening of the national health system, the other systems that tackle social determinants of health, and the national health research system to boost country's probability of attaining SDG3 by 2030.

ACKNOWLEDGMENTS

We are immensely grateful to *El Shaddai* for encouraging and sustaining us in the whole process of undertaking the study reported in this paper. RDKM is indebted to her doctoral supervisor's, Dr Flavia Senkubuge, Professor Charles Hongoro and Dr Joyce Shirinde of the University of Pretoria, for their encouragement and continued guidance. The views expressed in this paper are those of authors only and should not be attributed to any of the institutions they are currently affiliated to.

ETHICAL COMPLIANCE

The authors declare that they have no conflict of interest. The study did not receive funding from any source. The study did not involve experiments with either humans or animals. It also did not entail interviews with humans. The study analysis completely relied upon publicly available data from secondary sources. Therefore, it did not require ethical approval.

REFERENCES

[1] Southern African Development Community (SADC). The consolidated treaty of the Southern African Development Community. Gaborone: SADC, 2011.

[2] International Monetary Fund (IMF). World economic outlook database, January 2019. Washington, DC, IMF. URL: https://www.imf.org/external/pubs/ft/weo/2018/02/weodata/index.aspx.

[3] United Nations Development Programme (UNDP). Human development indices and indicators: 2018 statistical update. New York: UNDP, 2018.

[4] Global Burden of Disease Collaborative Network. Global Burden of Disease Study 2017 (GBD 2017) Results. Seattle: Institute for Health Metrics and Evaluation (IHME), 2018. URL: http://ghdx.healthdata.org/gbd-results-tool.

[5] Government of the Republic of Zambia. Zambia national health strategic plan 2017 – 2021. Lusaka: Ministry of Health, 2016.

[6] World Health Organization (WHO). The 2017 update, Global Health Workforce Statistics. Geneva: WHO, 2017.

[7] WHO. World health statistics overview 2019: Monitoring health for the SDGs, sustainable development goals. Geneva: WHO, 2019.

[8] WHO. Global Health Observatory data repository. Water, sanitation and hygiene. Geneva, WHO, 2019b. URL: http://apps.who.int/gho/data/node.main.46?lang=en.

[9] WHO. Global Health Expenditure Database. Geneva, WHO, 2019. URL: http://apps.who.int/nha/database/Select/Indicators/en.

[10] Stenberg K, Hanssen O, Edejer TT, Bertram M, Brindley C, Meshreky A, Rosen JE, Stover J, Verboom P, Sanders R, Soucat A. Financing transformative health systems towards achievement of the health sustainable development goals: A model for projected resource needs in 67 low-income and middle-income countries. Lancet Glob Health 2017;5:e875-87. URL: https://doi.org/10.1016/S2214-109X(17)30263-2.

[11] Pang T, Sadana R, Hanney S, Bhutta ZA, Hyder AA, Simon J. Knowledge for better health — a conceptual framework and foundation for health research systems. B World Health Organ 2003; 81:815-20.

[12] Kirigia JM, Ota MO, Senkubuge F, Wiysonge CS, Mayosi BM. Developing the African national health research systems barometer. Health Res Policy Sy 2016;14:53. URL: https://doi.org/10.1186/s12961-016-0121-4.

[13] 13.Rusakaniko S, Makanga M, Ota MO, Bockarie M, Banda G, Okeibunor J, Mutapi F, Tumusiime P, Nyirenda T, Kirigia JM, Nabyonga-Orem J. Strengthening national health research systems in the WHO African Region – progress towards universal health coverage. Globalization Health 2019; 15:50. URL: https://doi.org/10.1186/s12992-019-0492-8.

[14] Organization of African Unity (OAU). Abuja declaration on HIV/AIDS, tuberculosis and other related infectious diseases. Declaration OAU/SPS/Abuja/3. Addis Ababa: OAU, 2001a.

[15] Commission on Health Research for Development. Health research: Essential link to equity in development. New York: Oxford University Press, 1990.

[16] World Health Organization Regional Office for Africa (WHO/AFRO). Health financing: a strategy for the African region. Regional Committee for Africa resolution AFR/RC56/R5. Brazzaville: WHO/AFRO, 2006.

[17] Rice DP, Hodgson TA, Kopstein AN. The economic costs of illness: A replication and update. Health Care Financ Rev 1985;7(1):61-80.

[18] Brezinski EA, Dhillon JS, Armstrong AW. Economic Burden of Psoriasis in the United States: A Systematic Review. JAMA Dermatol 2015;151(6):651-8.

[19] Jiang R, Lee I, Lee TA, Pickard AS. The societal cost of heroin use disorder in the United States. PLoS One 2017;12(5):e0177323. URL: https://doi.org/10.1371/journal.pone.0177323.

[20] Robinson LS, Sarkies M, Brown T, O'Brien L. Direct, indirect and intangible costs of acute hand and wrist injuries: A systematic review. Injury 2016;47(12):2614–26.

[21] American Diabetes Association. Economic costs of diabetes in the U.S. in 2007. Diabetes Care 2008;31(3):596-615.

[22] Wu EQ, Birnbaum HG, Shi L, Ball DE, Kessler RC, Moulis M, Aggarwal J. The economic burden of schizophrenia in the United States in 2002. J Clin Psychiatry 2005;66(9):1122-9.

[23] Wolf AM, Colditz GA. Current estimates of the economic cost of obesity in the United States. Obes Res 1998;6(2):97-106.

[24] Sobocki P, Jönsson B, Angst J, Rehnberg C. Cost of depression in Europe. J Ment Health Policy Econ 2006;9(2):87-98.

[25] Pugliatti M1, Beghi E, Forsgren L, Ekman M, Sobocki P. Estimating the cost of epilepsy in Europe: a review with economic modeling. Epilepsia 2007;48(12):2224-33.

[26] Gustavsson A, Svensson M, Jacobi F, Allgulander C, Alonso J, Beghi E, Dodel R, Ekman M, Faravelli C, Fratiglioni L, et al. Cost of disorders of the brain in Europe 2010. Eur Neuropsychopharmacol 2011;21(10):718-79.

[27] Rotstein Z, Hazan R, Barak Y, Achiron A. Perspectives in multiple sclerosis health care: special focus on the costs of multiple sclerosis. Autoimmun Rev 2006;5(8):511-6.

[28] Chakravarthy U, Biundo E, Saka RO, Fasser C, Bourne R, Little JA. The economic impact of blindness in Europe. Ophthalmic Epidemiol 2017;24(4):239-47.

[29] Krensel M, Schäfer I, Augustin M. Cost-of-illness of melanoma in Europe - a systematic review of the published literature. J Eur Acad Dermatol Venereol 2019; 33(3):504-10.

[30] Brodszky V, Beretzky Z, Baji P, Rencz F, Péntek M, Rotar A, Tachkov K, Mayer S, Simon J, Niewada M, Hren R, Gulácsi L. Cost-of-illness studies in nine Central and Eastern European countries. Eur J Health Econ 2019;20(Suppl 1):155-72.

[31] Tack J, Stanghellini V, Mearin F, Yiannakou Y, Layer P, Coffin B, Simren M, Mackinnon J, Wiseman G, Marciniak A; IBIS-C Study group. Economic burden of moderate to severe irritable bowel syndrome with constipation in six European countries. BMC Gastroenterol 2019;19(1):69. URL: https://doi.org/10.1186/s12876-019-0985-1.

[32] Kirigia JM, Muthuri RDK, Nabyonga-Orem J, Kirigia DW. Counting the cost of child mortality in the World Health Organization African region. BMC Public Health 2015;15:1103. URL: https://doi.org/10.1186/s12889-015-2465-z.

[33] Kirigia JM, Masiye F, Kirigia DW, Akweongo P. Indirect costs associated with deaths from the Ebola virus disease in West Africa. Infect Dis Poverty 2015;4:45. URL: https://doi.org/10.1186/s40249-015-0079-4.

[34] Kirigia JM, Muthuri RDK: Productivity losses associated with tuberculosis deaths in the World Health Organization African Region. Infect Dis Poverty 2016;5:43. URL: https://doi.org/10.1186/s40249-016-0138-5.

[35] Kirigia JM, Mwabu GM, Orem JN, Muthuri RDK. Indirect cost of maternal deaths in the WHO African Region, 2013. Int J Soc Econ 2016;43(5):532-48.

[36] Kirigia JM, Mwabu GM, M'Imunya JM, Muthuri RDKM, Nkanata LHK, Gitonga EB. Indirect cost of non-communicable diseases deaths in the World Health Organization African Region. Int Arch Med 2017;10:34. URL: http://imedicalsociety.org/ojs/index.php/iam/article/view/2400/2057.

[37] Kirigia JM, Mburugu GN. The monetary value of human lives lost due to neglected tropical diseases in Africa. Infect Dis Poverty 2017; 6:165. URL: https://doi.org/10.1186/s40249-017-0379-y.

[38] WHO. A heavy burden: the productivity cost of illness in Africa. Brazzaville: WHO Regional Office for Africa, 2019.

[39] Kirigia JM, Mwabu GM. The monetary value of disability-adjusted-life-years lost in the East African community in 2015. Modern Economy 2018;9:1360-77.

[40] Muthuri RDK, Muthuri NG, Kirigia JM. Pecuniary value of disability-adjusted-life-years in the Arab Maghreb Union in 2015. J Hum Resource Sustain Stud 2018;6:249-74.

[41] Kirigia JM, Muthuri RNDK, Gitonga N. Fiscal value of disability-adjusted-life-years lost in the economic and monetary community of Central Africa (CEMAC). Int Public Health J 2019;11(2):155-83.

[42] The World Bank. World Development Report 1993 Investing in Health. Oxford: Oxford University Press, 1993.

[43] Murray CJL. Quantifying the burden of disease: the technical basis for disability-adjusted life years. Bull World Health Organ 1994;72(3):429-45.

[44] GBD 2017 DALYs and HALE Collaborators. Global, regional, and national disability-adjusted life years (DALYs) for 359 diseases and injuries and healthy life expectancy (HALE) for 195 countries and territories, 1990–2017: A systematic analysis for the Global Burden of Disease Study 2017. Lancet 2018;392:1859–1922.

[45] Weisbrod BA. The valuation of human capital. J Polit Econ 1961;69(5):425-36.

[46] UN. Transforming our world: The 2030 agenda for sustainable development. Seventieth session of the United Nations General Assembly Resolution A/RES/70/1. New York: UN, 2015.

[47] UNICEF. How to calculate average annual rate of reduction (AARR) of underweight prevalence. Statistics and Monitoring Section/Division of Policy and Practice Technical Note. New York: UNICEF, 2007.

[48] WHO. Global health sector strategy on HIV 2016-2021: Towards ending AIDS. The Sixty-Ninth World Health Assembly Document A69/31. Geneva: WHO, 2016.

[49] WHO. Global technical strategy for malaria 2016-2030. Geneva: WHO, 2015.

[50] WHO. World Mmalaria report 2018. Geneva: WHO, 2018.

[51] WHO. Global tuberculosis report 2018. Geneva: WHO, 2017.

[52] WHO. The end TB strategy. Geneva: WHO, 2015.

[53] WHO. Global vector control response 2017–2030. Geneva: WHO, 2017.

[54] WHO. Global health sector strategy on viral hepatitis, 2016–2021. Geneva: WHO, 2016.

[55] Government of the Republic of Zambia. Comprehensive immunization multi-year plan 2011-2015. Lusaka, Ministry of Health, 2011.

[56] Government of the Republic of Zambia. Reproductive, maternal, newborn, child and adolescent health and nutrition communication and advocacy strategy 2018-2021. Lusaka: Ministry of Health, 2018.

[57] Government of the Republic of Zambia. Zambia national maternal and neonatal services referral guidelines – Lusaka: Ministry of Health, 2018.

[58] Government of the Republic of Zambia. Adolescent Health Strategic Plan 2011 to 2015. Lusaka: Ministry of Health, 2011.

[59] Government of the Republic of Zambia. Zambia newborn health care framework. Lusaka: Ministry of Health, 2013.

[60] Government of the Republic of Zambia. National Food and Nutrition Strategic Plan for Zambia 2011-2015. Lusaka: National Food and Nutrition Commission of Zambia, 2011.

[61] Government of the Republic of Zambia. The National Health Services Act. Chapter 315 of The Laws of Zambia. Lusaka: Republic of Zambia, 1995.

[62] Government of the Republic of Zambia. The Medical and Allied Professions Act. Chapter 297 of The Laws of Zambia. Lusaka: Republic of Zambia, 1994.

[63] Government of the Republic of Zambia. The nurses and midwives bill, 2019. Lusaka: Republic of Zambia, 2019.

[64] Government of the Republic of Zambia. The Protection of Traditional Knowledge, Genetic Resources and Expressions of Folklore Act, 2016 No. 16 of the Laws of Zambia. Lusaka: Government of the Republic of Zambia, 2016.

[65] African Union (AU). Maputo plan of action for the operationalisation of the continental policy framework for sexual and reproductive health and rights 2007-2010. Doc. Sp/MIN/CAMH/5(I). Addis Ababa: AU, 2006.

[66] AU. Decision on the Report of the Implementation Status of Decision Assembly/AU/Dec.204 (XI) on Promotion of Maternal, Infant and Child Health and Development in Africa - Doc. Assembly/AU/6(XII). The Assembly of the African Union Twelfth Ordinary Session decision Assembly/AU/Dec.216(XII). Addis Ababa: AU, 2009.

[67] AU. Campaign for Accelerated Reduction of Maternal Mortality (CARMA). Addis Ababa: AU, 2009.

[68] AU. Actions on Maternal, New-born and Child Health and Development in Africa By 2015. Declaration Assembly/AU/Decl.1(XV) of the Assembly of the African Union Fifteenth Ordinary Session. Addis Ababa: AU, 2010.
[69] AU. Decision on the Reduction of Maternal, New-born and Child Mortality and Morbidity in Africa – Doc. Assembly/AU/12(XX)Add.4. The Assembly of the African Union Twentieth Ordinary Session decision Assembly/AU/Dec.461(XX). Addis Ababa: AU, 2013.
[70] AU. Declaration on Ending Preventable Child and Maternal Death in Africa – Doc. Assembly/AU/18(XXIII) Add.3. Assembly of The African Union Twenty-Third Ordinary Session decision Assembly/AU/Decl.2(XXIII). Addis Ababa: AU, 2014.
[71] AU. Decision on Progress on Maternal, New Born and Child Health (MNCH). 30th Ordinary Session of the Assembly decision Assembly/AU/Dec.680(XXX). Addis Ababa: AU, 2018.
[72] AU. Decision on Galvanizing Political Commitment Towards the Elimination of Female Genital Mutilation in Africa. The Assembly of the Union Thirty Second Ordinary Session decision Assembly/AU/Dec.737(XXXII). Addis Ababa: AU, 2019.
[73] AU. Declaration on Addressing Social Determinants of Health in Africa: Adoption of Health in All Policies Approach. The Assembly of The Union Thirty Second Ordinary Session declaration Assembly/AU/Decl.3(XXXII). Addis Ababa: AU, 2019.
[74] United Nations (UN). Human Rights Council Preventable Maternal Mortality and Morbidity and Human Rights A/HRC/11/L.16/Rev 1. New York: UN, 2009.
[75] UN. Preventable maternal mortality and morbidity and human rights. United Nations General Assembly (UNGA) resolution A/HRC/33/L.3/Rev.1. New York: UN, 2016.
[76] UN. Report of the Office of the United Nations High Commissioner for Human Rights on preventable maternal mortality and morbidity and human rights. UNGA resolution A/HRC/14/39. New York: Human Rights Council, 2010.
[77] UN. Elimination of preventable maternal mortality and morbidity and the empowerment of women. Commission on the Status of Women resolution E/CN.6/2011/CRP.8. New York: UN, 2011.
[78] UN. Intensification of efforts to end obstetric fistula. UNGA resolution A/RES/71/169. New York: UN, 2017.
[79] UN. Intensification of efforts to prevent and eliminate all forms of violence against women and girls: domestic violence. UNGA resolution A/RES/71/170. New York: UN, 2017.
[80] UN. Rights of the child. UNGA resolution A/RES/71/177. New York: UN, 2017.
[81] UN. Child, early and forced marriage. UNGA resolution A/RES/71/175. New York: UN, 2017.
[82] UN. Intensifying global efforts for the elimination of female genital mutilation. UNGA resolution A/RES/73/149. New York: UN, 2018.

[83] UN. Intensification of efforts to prevent and eliminate all forms of violence against women and girls: sexual harassment. UNGA resolution A/RES/73/148. New York: UN, 2018.

[84] WHO. Working towards the reduction of perinatal and neonatal mortality. Sixty-fourth World Health Assembly resolution WHA64.13. Geneva: WHO, 2011.

[85] WHO. Ending inappropriate promotion of foods for infants and young children. Sixty-ninth World Health Assembly resolution WHA69.9. Geneva: WHO, 2016.

[86] WHO. United Nations Decade of Action on Nutrition (2016–2025). Sixty-ninth World Health Assembly resolution WHA69.8. Geneva: WHO, 2016.

[87] WHO. Infant and young child feeding. Seventy-First World Health Assembly resolution WHA71.9. Geneva: WHO, 2018.

[88] WHO. Global vaccine action plan. Sixty-eighth World Health Assembly resolution WHA68.6. Geneva: WHO, 2015.

[89] WHO. Strengthening immunization to achieve the goals of the global vaccine action plan. Seventieth World Health Assembly Resolution WHA70.14. Geneva: WHO, 2017.

[90] WHO. Promoting innovation and access to quality, safe, efficacious and affordable medicines for children. Sixty-ninth World Health Assembly resolution WHA69.20. Geneva: WHO, 2016.

[91] WHO. Committing to implementation of the Global Strategy for Women's, Children's and Adolescents' Health. Sixty-ninth World Health Assembly resolution WHA69.2. Geneva: WHO, 2016f.

[92] WHO. WHO global plan of action to strengthen the role of the health system within a national multi-sectoral response to address interpersonal violence, in particular against women and girls, and against children. Sixty-ninth World Health Assembly resolution WHA69.5. Geneva: WHO, 2016.

[93] WHO. Strengthening integrated, people-centred health services. Sixty-ninth World Health Assembly resolution WHA69.24. Geneva: WHO, 2016.

[94] Government of the Republic of Zambia. National HIV/AIDS/STI/TB Policy. Lusaka, Ministry of Health, 2002a.

[95] Government of the Republic of Zambia. HIV and AIDS policy for the transport sector in ZAMBIA. Lusaka: Ministry of Communications and Transport, 2010.

[96] Government of the Republic of Zambia. A comprehensive HIV prevention roadmap 2017-2021: framework of indicators and targets. Lusaka: National HIV/AIDS/STI/TB Council, 2017.

[97] Government of the Republic of Zambia. National Malaria Elimination Strategic Plan (NMESP) 2017–2021. Lusaka, Ministry of Health, 2017.

[98] Government of the Republic of Zambia. Ministry of Health elimination of neglected tropical diseases national masterplan 2019 – 2023. Lusaka: Ministry of Health, 2019.

[99] Government of the Republic of Zambia. Public Health Act. Chapter 295 of The Laws of Zambia. Lusaka: Ministry of Health, 1995.

[100] Government of the Republic of Zambia. National HIV/AIDS/STI/TB Council Act No. 10 of 2002. Lusaka: Republic of Zambia, 2002.

[101] OAU. OAU. Decision on the African Summit on HIV / AIDS, Tuberculosis and Other Related Infectious Diseases. Decision AHG / Dec.161 (XXXVII) of the 37th Ordinary Session of the Conference of Heads of State and Government. Addis Ababa: OAU, 2001.

[102] AU. Decision on the continental framework for harmonization of approaches among member states, and integration of policies on human rights and people infected and affected by HIV/AIDS in Africa. DOC.ASSEMBLY/AU/5 (VII). Decision Assembly/AU/Dec.116(VII) of the Assembly of the African Union Seventh Ordinary Session. Addis Ababa: AU, 2006.

[103] AU. Decision on Abuja call for accelerated action towards universal access to HIV/AIDS, tuberculosis and malaria (ATM) services in Africa. DOC.ASSEMBLY/AU/5 (VII). Decision Assembly/AU/Dec.115 (VII) of the Assembly of the African Union Seventh Ordinary Session. Addis Ababa: AU, 2006.

[104] AU. Decision on the Five (5)-Year Review of the Abuja Call for Accelerated Action Towards Universal Access to HIV/AIDS, Tuberculosis and Malaria Services in Africa. Doc. EX.CL/592(XVII). The Assembly of the African Union Fifteenth Ordinary Session Decision Assembly/AU/Dec.291(XV). Addis Ababa: AU, 2010.

[105] AU. Declaration on the Report of AIDS Watch Africa (AWA) Action Committee of Heads of State and Government. Assembly of the Union Nineteenth Ordinary Session Declaration Assembly/AU/Decl. 2(XIX). Addis Ababa: AU, 2012.

[106] WHO. Global health sector strategies on HIV, viral hepatitis and sexually transmitted infections, for the period 2016–2021. Sixty-ninth World Health Assembly resolution WHA69.22. Geneva: WHO, 2016.

[107] WHO. Global technical strategy and targets for malaria 2016–2030. Sixty-eighth World Health Assembly resolution WHA68.2. Geneva: WHO, 2015.

[108] WHO. Global vector control response: an integrated approach for the control of vector-borne diseases. Seventieth World Health Assembly Resolution WHA70.16. Geneva: WHO, 2017.

[109] UN. Political Declaration on HIV and AIDS: On the Fast Track to Accelerating the Fight against HIV and to Ending the AIDS Epidemic by 2030. UNGA resolution A/RES/70/266. New York: UN, 2016.

[110] UN. Scope, modalities, format and organization of the high-level meeting on the fight against tuberculosis. UNGA resolution A/RES/72/268. New York: UN, 2018.

[111] UN. Political declaration of the high-level meeting of the General Assembly on antimicrobial resistance. UNGA resolution A/RES/71/3. New York: UN, 2016.

[112] UN. Consolidating gains and accelerating efforts to control and eliminate malaria in developing countries, particularly in Africa, by 2030. UNGA resolution A/RES/72/309. New York: UN, 2018.

[113] UN. The human rights to safe drinking water and sanitation. United Nations General Assembly Resolution A/RES/72/178. New York: UN, 2017.

[114] Government of the Republic of Zambia. Zambian Strategic Plan 2013-2016: non-communicable diseases and their risk factors. Lusaka: Ministry of Health, 2013b.

[115] Government of the Republic of Zambia. National cancer control strategic plan 2016-2021. Lusaka: Ministry of Health, 2016c.

[116] Government of the Republic of Zambia. National health in all policies strategic framework 2017-2021. Lusaka: Ministry of Health, 2018.

[117] Government of the Republic of Zambia. The Mental Health Act, 2019. Lusaka: Zambia, 2019.

[118] Government of the Republic of Zambia. Chapter 311 Ionising Radiation Protection Act. Act 16 of 2005, Act 19 of 2011, Act 119 of 2006. Lusaka: Republic of Zambia, 2011.

[119] Government of the Republic of Zambia. The Occupational Health and Safety Act, 2010. Lusaka: Zambia, 2010.

[120] WHO. Prevention and control of noncommunicable diseases. Fifty-third World Health Assembly resolution WHA53.17. Geneva: WHO, 2000.

[121] WHO. Framework convention on tobacco control. Fifty-third World Health Assembly resolution WHA53.16. Geneva: WHO, 2000.

[122] WHO. Strategies to reduce the harmful use of alcohol. Sixty-first World Health Assembly resolution WHA61.4. Geneva: WHO, 2008.

[123] WHO. Prevention and control of noncommunicable diseases: implementation of the global strategy. Sixty-first World Health Assembly resolution WHA61.14. Geneva: WHO, 2008.

[124] WHO. Follow-up to the Political Declaration of the High-level Meeting of the General Assembly on the Prevention and Control of Noncommunicable Diseases. Sixty-sixth World Health Assembly resolution WHA66.10. Geneva: WHO, 2013.

[125] WHO. Global action plan for the prevention and control of noncommunicable diseases 2013–2020. Sixty-sixth World Health Assembly doc. A66/9. Geneva: WHO, 2013.

[126] WHO. Comprehensive mental health action plan 2013–2020. Sixty-sixth World Health Assembly resolution WHA66.8. Geneva: WHO, 2013.

[127] WHO. Towards universal eye health: a global action plan 2014–2019. Sixty-sixth World Health Assembly resolution WHA66.4. Geneva: WHO, 2013.

[128] WHO. Health and the environment: addressing the health impact of air pollution. Sixty-eighth World Health Assembly resolution WHA68.8. Geneva: WHO, 2015.

[129] WHO. Global strategy and action plan on ageing and health 2016–2020: towards a world in which everyone can live a long and healthy life. Sixty-ninth World Health Assembly resolution WHA69.3. Geneva: WHO, 2016.

[130] WHO. Cancer prevention and control in the context of an integrated approach. Seventieth World Health Assembly Resolution WHA70.12. Geneva: WHO, 2017.

[131] WHO. Global action plan on the public health response to dementia. Seventieth World Health Assembly Resolution WHA70(17). Geneva: WHO, 2017.

[132] WHO. WHO global action plan on physical activity 2018–2030. Seventy-First World Health Assembly resolution WHA71.6. Geneva: WHO; 2018.

[133] UN. Political Declaration of the High-level Meeting of the General Assembly on the Prevention and Control of Noncommunicable Diseases. UNGA resolution A/RES/66/2. New York: UN, 2012.

[134] UN. Scope, modalities, format and organization of the third high-level meeting of the General Assembly on the Prevention and Control of Non-Communicable Diseases. UNGA resolution A/RES/72/274. New York: UN, 2018.

[135] UN. Follow-up to the Second World Assembly on Ageing. UNGA resolution A/RES/72/144. New York: UN, 2017.

[136] UN. Implementation of the United Nations Decade of Action on Nutrition (2016-2025). UNGA resolution A/RES/72/306. New York: UN, 2018.

[137] Government of the Republic of Zambia. National Road Safety Policy Strategy and Action Plan 2020. Lusaka: Zambia Road Safety Agency, 2016.

[138] Government of the Republic of Zambia Republic Zambia. Road Traffic Act No. 11 of 2002. Lusaka: Government of the Republic of Zambia Republic Zambia, 2002.

[139] WHO. Addressing the challenges of the United Nations Decade of Action for Road Safety (2011–2020): outcome of the second Global High-level Conference on Road Safety – Time for Results. Sixty-ninth World Health Assembly resolution WHA69.7. Geneva: WHO, 2016.

[140] UN. Improving global road safety. UNGA resolution A/RES/64/255. New York: UN, 2010.

[141] UN. Improving global road safety. UNGA resolution A/RES/66/260. New York: UN, 2012.

[142] UN. Improving global road safety. UNGA resolution A/RES/68/269. New York: UN, 2014.

[143] UN. Improving global road safety. UNGA resolution A/RES/70/260.New York: UNI, 2016.

[144] UN. Improving global road safety. UNGA resolution A/RES/70/260.New York: UN, 2018.

[145] GBD 2017 Mortality Collaborators. Global, regional, and national age-sex-specific mortality and life expectancy, 1950–2017: A systematic analysis for the Global Burden of Disease Study 2017. Lancet 2018;392:1684–735.

[146] GBD 2017 DALYs and HALE Collaborators. Global, regional, and national disability-adjusted life-years (DALYs) for 359 diseases and injuries and healthy life expectancy (HALE) for 195 countries and territories, 1990–2017: a systematic analysis for the Global Burden of Disease Study 2017. Lancet 2018;392:1859–1922.

[147] GBD 2017 Disease and Injury Incidence and Prevalence Collaborators. Global, regional, and national incidence, prevalence, and years lived with disability for 354 diseases and injuries for 195 countries and territories, 1990–2017: a systematic analysis for the Global Burden of Disease Study 2017. Lancet 2018; 92:1789–1858.

[148] Giannetti BF, Agostinho F, Almeida CMVB, Huisingh D. A review of limitations of GDP and alternative indices to monitor human wellbeing and to manage eco-system functionality. J Clean Prod 2015;87:11-25.

In: Disability: International Aspects
Editors: Ariel Tenenbaum et al.
ISBN: 978-1-53617-886-9

Chapter 15

Disability in North Africa: Prevalence, Pattern, and Recommendations

Miracle A Adesina*[1,2] *and Kehinde K Kanmodi*[2-5,*]*, BDS
[1]Department of Physiotherapy, University of Ibadan, Ibadan, Nigeria
[2]Cephas Health Research Initiative Inc, Ibadan, Nigeria
[3]Dental Clinic, Kebbi Medical Centre, Kalgo, Nigeria
[4]National Teachers' Institute, Kaduna, Nigeria
[5]Department of Political Science,
National Open University of Nigeria, Abuja, Nigeria

Abstract

Disability can be described as a condition encapsulating impairments, activity limitation and participation restriction. This chapter aims to do a comparative analysis on the prevalence, socio-demographic distribution and distribution patterns of disability among the people living in the member nations of the northern region of Africa. Methods: This study

---

* Corresponding Author: Kehinde K Kanmodi, BDS, Department of Political Science, National Open University of Nigeria, Abuja, Nigeria. E-mail: kanmodikehinde@yahoo.com.

was an original research conducted on the population of people living with disability in North Africa. Secondary data obtained from the most recent national housing and population surveys released by the statistics bureau of the member countries of the northern region of Africa were utilized for this study. Results: The findings from this study reveals that Libya has the highest prevalence rate of disabled (5.8%); Sudan has the highest population of disabled (1,854,985); Algeria has the highest disabled male population (1,300,689); and Sudan has the highest disabled children population (387,692). The pattern of disability follows a decreasing trend from physical to speech disability. Conclusions: Disability is a major problem of global health importance in North Africa. There is an imminent need for the governments of the North Africa nations to look into this health problem in their region.

INTRODUCTION

Disability is an umbrella term, covering impairments, activity limitations and participation restriction. To start with: impairment can be described as a problem in body function or structure; activity limitation means a difficulty encountered by an individual in executing a task or action; and participation restriction refers to a problem experienced by an individual in involvement in life situations (1). Disability issues are of global health concern, as its impacts have far reaching effects on the quality of life of people living with such condition (2).

There are "reliable" statistics on the prevalence rates and some socio-demographic distribution of people living with disability in the member countries that make up North Africa region (2-8), but very few scientific publications on the disability attributes in this region (9-14). However, virtually all publications available on disability studies in this region presented information only on the individual member nations – Algeria (15), Egypt (16), Libya (17), Morocco (18), Sudan (19) and Tunisia (20).

There is virtually no literature comparing disability statistics across the member nations of the northern Africa region; this shows the need to conduct a study to look into the global prevalence as well as the socio-demographic distribution of disability in the northern region of Africa. A study conducted on this area will help scientific researchers, policy makers, governmental bodies, and other stake holders in the formulation, review, and execution of policy that will adequately cater for the needs of the people living with disability in this geographical region of Africa. The outcomes of such study conducted on this policy research area will also go a long way in the improvement of the quality of life of people living with disability in this delimitated geographical region.

This study aims to: do a comparative analysis on the prevalence rates of disability; determine the socio-demographic distribution of people living with disability; and also determine the distribution patterns of disability among the people living in the member nations of the northern region of Africa.

OUR STUDY

This study was an original research conducted on the population of people living with disability in North Africa. Secondary data obtained from the most recent national housing and population surveys released by the statistics bureau of the member countries of the northern region of Africa were utilized for this study. The member countries of the North Africa region are Algeria, Egypt, Libya, Morocco, Sudan, Tunisia, and Western Sahara (21). The secondary data on disability that were utilized for this study were obtained from the following sources:

1. Office Nationale des Statistiques (National Bureau of Statistics), Algeria (2006).
2. 2006 Population and Housing Census, Egypt, (2006).
3. National Libya Family Health Survey, (2007).
4. National Survey on Disability, Morocco, (2014)
5. 2008 Population and Housing Census, Sudan, (2008).
6. 2009 Population and Housing Census, Tunisia, (2009).

Data on the prevalence rate of disability, sex distribution of people living with disability, distribution of disability among children, as well as the pattern of distribution of different forms of disability in the countries in the southern region of Africa were extracted from the above listed databases. Data analysis was done using the Microsoft Excel Version 2011. Presentation of the findings was done in sentences, tables, and charts.

FINDINGS

The findings made from the analysis of the secondary data obtained for each of the northern African countries are relayed as follows:

Table 1. Prevalence of disability in North Africa

Country	Population with disability	Population without disability	Total population	Prevalence of disability
Algeria	1,667,550	31,603,450	33,351,000	5%
Egypt	475,576	72,322,455	72,798,031	0.7%
Libya	312,813	5,080,512	5,393,325	5.8%
Morocco	1,703,424	31,697,047	33,460,471	5.1%
Sudan	1,854,985	36,349,975	38,204,690	4.9%
Tunisia	140.026	10,280,425	10,420,451	1.3%

Algeria

The estimated prevalence rate of disability in Algeria, based on the data released by the National Bureau of Statistics in Algeria, in the year 2006, was 5% (1,667,550/33,351,000) (see Table 1). The pattern of gender distribution of people living with disability is shown in Table 2: an estimated 1,300,689 males out of 16,808,904 males and 366,801 females of 16,542,096 females in Algeria are living with disability; this gives the estimated prevalence rate of 3.9% and 1.1% among males and females respectively. Statistics on the number of children in Algeria with disabilities and also the distribution of the different forms of disability was not obtained.

Table 2. Sex distribution of disability in North Africa

	Population with disability	Population without disability	Population with disability	Population without disability
Algeria	1,300,689	15,508,215	366,861	16,175,235
Egypt	305,216	36,913,840	170,360	35,408,615
Libya	134,833	2,578,009	177,980	2,464,749
Morocco	843,459	N/A	859,965	N/A
Sudan	968,086	18,353,885	886,899	17,996,100
Tunisia	89,156	5,125,289	50,870	5,155,136

N/A: Not available.

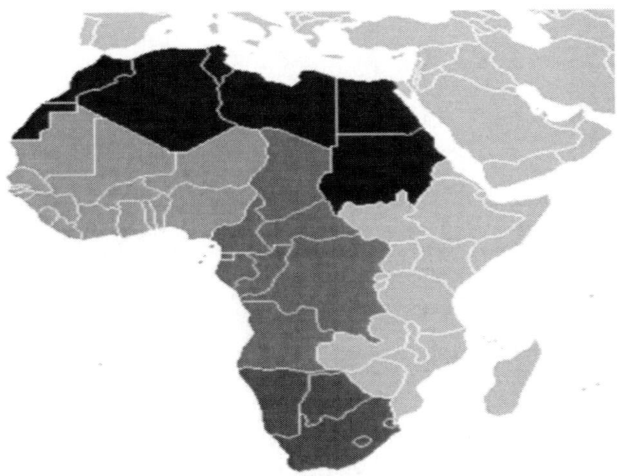

Source: Wikipedia.

Figure 1. Map showing North Africa (Colour blue).

Egypt

The prevalence rate of disability in Egypt, according to the 2006 Housing and Population Census in Egypt is depicted in Table 1. There are an estimated 475,576 people living with disability, out of a total population of 72,798,031, in Egypt; this figure gives the estimated prevalence rate as 0.7% for the total population. The sex distribution of those people living with disability in Egypt is presented in Table 2. Of the 35,578,975 females in Egypt, 170,360 are living with disability; and of the 37,219,056 total males, 305,216 of them are living with disability: this gives an estimated female prevalence of 0.5% and a male prevalence of 0.8%.

Table 3. Distribution of disability among children in North Africa

Country	Age range	Male with disability	Female with disability
Egypt	0 -14	32,315	39,497
Libya	0 – 14	27,134	30,111
Sudan	0 – 15	200,824	186,868
Tunisia	0 - 15	89,156	50,870

Statistics on the number of children with disabilities within the age range 0 – 14 years are also given in the 2006 census. A total of 71,812 children are living with disability, of which 55% of them are females (see Table 3).

Table 4 depicts the pattern of disability among the people in Egypt. Of those individuals living with disability, 13.3% of them had sight or visual impairment (blind and one-eyed), 33.9% had physical impairment (impairment of leg(s), impairment of hand(s), infantile paralysis and total or partial paralysis), 6.6%% had both visual and speech impairment, 22.4% had mental impairment, 3.5% had hearing impairment, 2.6% had speech impairment, and 17.7% had other forms of disability which were not classified.

Libya

With reference to the National Libya Family Health Survey in 2007, the prevalence rate of disability in Libya is 5.8% (see Table 1). The distribution of disability between male and female is displayed in Table 2: 177,980 of the females in Libya are estimated to be living with disability (giving a prevalence disability rate of 3.3% among women) while 134,833 males are living with disability, giving a prevalence disability rate of 2.5% among males.

Table 4. Prevalence of forms of disabilities in North Africa

Country	Forms of Disability											
	Visual	Mobility/ Physical	Visual & Speech	Mental	Hearing	Communication/ Speech	Self-Care	Impairment in socialising	Remembering	Speech & Hearing	Others	Multiple
Egypt	13.3%	33.9%	6.6%	22.4%	3.5%	2.6%	NA	NA	NA	NA	17.7%	NA
Libya	11.8%	28.5%	NA	NA	16.3%	22.5%	14.5%	48.3%	NA	NA	NA	NA
Morocco	7.5%	4.9%	NA	NA	3.5%	1.5%	2.3%	NA	1.5%	NA	NA	NA
Sudan	36.5%	28.5%	NA	24.2%	16.6%	6.4%	NA	NA	NA	NA	NA	NA
Tunisia	10%	36.7%	NA	0.34%	0.05%	4.7%	NA	NA	NA	3.7%	NA	5.8%

Out of the total number of children in Libya within the age range of 0 – 14 years (57,245), 52.6% (30,111) are females and 47.4% (27,134) are males (see Table 3).

Less than one-third (28.5%) of individuals with disability have mobility/physical impairment, visual impairment (11.8%), hearing impairment (16.3%), speech and communication impairments (22.5%), self-care impairment (14.8%) and impairment in socializing (48.3%) (See Table 4).

Morocco

The prevalence rate of disability in Morocco is shown in Table 1. As at 2014, there are about 1,703,424 people living with disability out of a total population of about 33,400,471 people in this country. By mathematical implication, the prevalence rate of disability in Morocco is 5.1%.

Statistics also revealed that 859,965 females in Morocco are living with disability and 843,459 males living in Morocco have disability (see Table 2).

The estimated number of children with disability within age range of 0 to 15 years is 6,863. This is depicted in Table 3. It is also observed that 7.5% of individuals living in Morocco had seeing impairment, 1.5% had remembering impairment, 3.5% had hearing impairment, 4.9% had walking impairment, 2.3% had self-care impairment, and 1.5% had communication impairment (see Table 4).

Sudan

The prevalence rate of disability in Swaziland, based on the 2008 Housing and Population Census in Sudan, was 4.9% (see Table 1). The pattern of gender distribution of people living with disability is depicted in Table 3: the prevalence rates of disability among males and females in Sudan were 5.0% and 4.7% respectively.

Statistics on the number of children in Sudan with disabilities within the range of age 0 – 14 years are presented in Table 3. An estimated number of 387,692 children within age range 0 – 14 years are living with disability, of which 200,824 are males and 186,868 are females.

Table 4 depicts the pattern of distribution of the forms of disability among the people living in Sudan: less than four-tenth (36.5%) of the individuals with disability in Sudan had visual impairment; 16.6% of had hearing impairment; 6.4% had speech impairment; 24.2% had mental impairment; and 28.5% had physical impairment.

Tunisia

With reference to the 2009 Population and Housing Census in Tunisia, the prevalence rate of disability in Tunisia is 1.3%. The distribution of disability between male and female is displayed in Table 2: 50,870 out of the 5,206,006 total Tunisia female population are estimated to be living with disability (giving a prevalence disability rate of 1.0% among women) while 89,156 out of the 5,214,445 total Tunisia male population are living with disability, giving a prevalence disability rate of 1.7% among males. Out of the total population of children within the age range of 0 – 14 years (14,283), 6,099 are males and 8,184 are females (Table 3).

It is also observed that: 10% of individuals living in Tunisia had visual impairment, 34.1% had mental impairment, 5.1% had hearing impairment, 36.7% had physical impairment, 4.7% had speech impairment, 3.7% had both speech and hearing impairment and 5.8% had multiple impairments (Table 4).

Western Sahara

No data on disability in Western Sahara was found.

Discussion

The estimated prevalence rates of disability in the member countries of the northern region of Africa ranges from 0.7-5.8%, with the lowest prevalence rate recorded in Egypt and highest rate recorded in Libya. This value is quite lower than the United States of America (11.9% in 2010; 12.6% in 2013, 2014 & 2015) (22). The total number of people living with disability in North African countries ranges from 86,874 to 1,854,985 people per country. Sudan has a lower prevalence rate of people living with disability than Libya; she (Sudan) also has the highest number of people living with disability in the northern region of Africa (1,854,985 people). Moreover, the statistics in this present study showed that Egypt has more people living with disability than Libya (475,576 versus 312,813).These numerical values that were obtained in North Africa populations is quite lower that recorded in Great Britain (11.2 million people in 2010/2011; 11.6 million people in 2011/2012) (23).

The gender distribution of people living with disability in the North Africa is discussed in this paragraph. The total number of males living with disability ranges from 89,156 (lowest in Tunisia) to 1,300,689 (highest in Algeria). Based on the data used for this present study, the sum total of the males and females living with disability in North Africa are 3,641,439 and 2,512,935 respectively; this gives a population difference of over 1,000,000 between both genders. This shows that more males are living with disability in North Africa. However, this finding is not consistent with what was recorded in Great Britain where there were more females than males with disabilities (with difference of about 900,000 in 2011/2012) and Southern Africa with a difference of over 500,000 (23, 24).

The total number of children, within the age range of 0 to 14 years, living with disability in the North African countries range from 14,283 (lowest in Tunisia) to 387,692 (highest in Sudan). It was observed that Sudan alone has 73% of children (0-14 years) living with disability in North Africa. The total number of male children within 0-14 years age range, who are living with disability, is lowest in Libya (27, 134) and highest in Sudan (200,824). Likewise, the total female children population with disability within the 0-14 years age group is lowest in Libya (30,111) and highest in Sudan (186,868). The total male population and female children population living with disability are 349,429 and 307,346 respectively; this gives a difference of more than 40,000 between the two genders. Hence, a higher proportion of the male children in North Africa are living with disability when compared with the female children.

Patterns of disability (focusing on impairment and activity limitation) in North Africa Disability is a condition covering impairments, activity limitations and participation restriction. The three component involved in defining disability are "impairment" which is "problem in body function and structure"; "activity limitation" which means "difficulty in executing task"; and "participation restriction" which means "problem encountered in involvement in life situations" (1). In the recent census survey conducted by the government of the North African nations, information on both impairment and activity limitation were obtained; however, participation restriction was not accessed as measures used in assessing disability in census surveys cover only impairments and activity limitation (25).

There were five patterns of disability that were measured in the population surveys used for this study: [1] visual disability; [2] hearing disability; [3] speech disability; [4] physical/walking/arm and leg disability and [5] mental disability. About 7.5% and 36.5% of people suffer from visual disability, in Morocco and in Sudan, respectively. However, in other member countries in North Africa, like Tunisia, Libya, and Egypt, about 10%, 11.8%, and 13.3% of their people are suffering from visual impairment. The pattern here is similar to what exists in Southern Africa region where about 1.8% to 35% of the population has visual disability (24). However, this finding is higher than that of United States (6.4% in 2008-10, 6.5% in 2011-12, 6.6% in 2013&2015, 6.7% in 2014) (22).

Census statistics also shows that about 0.05% of people in Tunisia and 16.6% in Sudan suffer from hearing disability. The findings for other nations in this region are: 3.5% (Egypt), 3.9% (Morocco) and 16.3% (Libya). The finding from census reveals that about 1.5% of people in Morocco and up to 22.5% in Libya have hearing disability. However, in Egypt, Tunisia and Sudan, about 2.6%, 4.7% and 6.4% of their people suffer from hearing disability. This finding here is quite similar to what obtains in Southern Africa region, where about 4.1% to 21% of people have hearing disability (24). However, the percentage of people with hearing disability for most North African countries is higher that want obtains in the United States (3.4% in 2009-12, 3.6% in 2013-15) (22).

It is of note that about 4.9% of people in Morocco and also about 36.7% in Tunisia have physical/walking/arm and leg disability. The occurrence in the other member countries in the northern region of Africa is 4.9% (Morocco), 28.5% (Libya), 28.5% (Sudan) and 33.9% (Egypt). Also, about 0.34% of persons in Tunisia, 6.6% in Egypt and 24.20% in Sudan suffer from mental disability. This is also consistent with findings from Southern Africa region where an estimated 1.7% to 37% of persons suffer from physical disability (24). However, this findings in not consistent with that of USA as most of the North Africa nations have higher percentage of people with walking disability (USA statistics: 4.6% in 2011-12, 4.7 in 2013 & 4.8% in 2014-15) (22), and also Great Britain (Great Britain statistics: 6.3% in 2002/03, 2007/08 & 2009/10; 6.2% in 2003/04, 2005-07; 6.4% in 2008/09 & 2010/11 and 6.5% in 2011/12) (23). In addition, an estimated 0.34% of people in Tunisia, 6.6% in Egypt and up to 24.20% in Sudan suffer from mental disability.

From the above, the average global prevalence rate of visual, hearing, speech, mental, physical/walking/arm and leg impairment in North Africa could be determined statistically. Hence, the average population size with visual impairment is 15.8%, hearing impairment (8.1%), speech impairment (7.54%), mental impairment (10.4%) and physical/walking/arm and leg impairment (44.2%). Physical/walking disability has the highest occurrence followed by visual disability, mental disability, hearing disability and speech disability, in decreasing order of frequency. Our finding is partially consistent with findings from USA, where walking disability was the most prevalent form of disability among her population; however, the total population of people with walking disability in the USA is lower than that recorded in each of the North Africa nations (22). It was also observed that Sudan had the highest population size of visual, hearing and mental impairment. This is however, not consistent with findings from the Southern Africa study where the most occurring disability is visual followed by physical, hearing and speech, in decreasing order of frequency (24).

Limitations of the study

This study involved the use of secondary data for analysis. Hence, the study has its peculiar limitations. Below are the limitations of this study in highlights:

- All of the available statistical data used for this study are older than three years, with the most recent data collected in the year 2014. This might not be consistent with present finding as this might be affected by variation in birth and death rate, immigration and emigration rate coupled with other factors.
- Statistics from Housing and Population Census sometimes cannot be completely trusted as they can be manipulated for political reasons, where results are altered by political leaders to increase financial allocation and provision to their area. However, data from census are still the best source of statistics for a study looking at a nation as an entity.
- Lack of uniform definition and classification of disability by the national census and bureau of statistics in the member nations of North Africa.

Recommendations

The following are recommendations made by the authors of this study to the government, policy makers, disability advocacy groups, non-governmental organization and other organizations:

- The government of the member nations of North Africa (Algeria, Egypt, Morocco Tunisia and Sudan) should set up a body to obtain regular statistics and data relating to people living with disability. This is a solution to the availability of old data and also because census cannot be advised to be too frequent as it is very expensive to do. The presence of this data will help and guide in provision of services and products for individuals with disability.
- Government and other bodies should make sure all public and private facilities are accessible to individuals with physical disabilities and also appropriate changes should be made to the transportation system so that transportation for them would be easy and stress-free. Also, more centers and facilities specialized for rehabilitation of the physically disabled should be set up.
- Government and other bodies should set up a body taking charge of their care. Intervention programs such as free eye glasses schemes, subsidized/free eye surgery programs, etc. can be set up. Also, other populations groups with disabilities other than visual impairment should not be neglected because they have smaller population size. The Equatorial Guinea experience can be adopted in this strategy, where the Ministry of Health, Equatorial Guinea, gave out wheelchairs to the physically disabled (26).
- Government and other bodies should provide equipment and facilities which will bring about better and enjoyable education for the disabled. The Cameroonian government operated a free education program for the individuals with disability (27); this can be adopted for use in North Africa.

CONCLUSION

Disability is a condition that affects an individual which might not be caused by the person affected. The society should not view disabled individuals as been unnecessary burden but as important component of the society. Result from this study shows that the estimated total number of people with disability in North Africa range from 86,874 to 1,854,985. Also, there are more males than females with disability (difference of more than 1,000,000) in this region. More than 600,000 children are living with disability in North Africa. Physical impairment is the most prevalent form of disability in North Africa. Individuals with disabilities are popularly known to have lifetime experience of social stigma, discrimination, lack of education, transportation and good health services, or inadequate access to public and private facility (9, 16, 27). Appropriate, practical, and feasible recommendations have been made in this study; the recommendations in this study will guide policy makers and executives in policy making and in the provision of services and facilities for the disabled individuals in North Africa.

Acknowledgments

Authors have no competing interest to declare. This study was self-funded.

References

[1] WHO. Disabilities. URL: www.who.int/topics/disabilities/en/.

[2] Hosain GM, Atkinson D, Underwood P. Impact of disability on quality of life of rural disabled people in Bangladesh J Health Popul Nutr 2002;20(4):297-305.

[3] Office Nationale des Statistiques, Algiers. Enquête nationale à indicateurs multiples (MICS), 2006. Cited by Economic and Social Commission of Western Asia (ESCWA) and League of Arab States 2014. URL: https://www.unescwa.org/sites/www.unescwa.org/files/page_attachments/disability_in_the_arab_region-_an_overview_-_en_1.pdf.

[4] Central Agency for Public Mobilization and Statistics, Cairo, Egypt. Population and Housing Census, 2006. Cited by Economic and Social Commission of Western Asia (ESCWA) and League of Arab States. URL: https://www.unescwa.org/sites/www.unescwa.org/files/page_attachments/disability_in_the_arab_region-_an_overview_-_en_1.pdf.

[5] Pan Arab Project for Family Health and the National Centre for Infectious and Chronic Disease Control. National Libyan Family Health Survey, 2007. Tripoli.

Cited by Economic and Social Commission of Western Asia (ESCWA) and League of Arab States. URL: https://www.unescwa.org/sites/www.unescwa.org/files/page_attachments/disability_in_the_arab_region-_an_overview_-_en_1.pdf.

[6] National Survey of Disability Morocco 2014. Cited by Lkhouf N. Disability statistics from the 2014 Moroccan census. High Commission for planning. Accessed 2018 Aug 01 URL: https://www.google.com/url?q=https://unstats.un,org/unsd/demographic-social/meetings/2017/oman--disabiliyu-measurement-and-statistics/Session%25206/Morocco.pdf&sa=U&ved=2ahUKEwi6pt-foMDcAhUI66QKHcuBDDgQFjAAegQIAAxAB&usg=AOvVaw3K-s9JyQgPQJVoNX4Octg.

[7] Central Bureau of Statistics. Fifth Population and Housing Census 2008. Khartoum. Cited by Economic and Social Commission of Western Asia (ESCWA) and League of Arab States. URL: https://www.unescwa.org/sites/www.unescwa.org/files/page_attachments/disability_in_the_arab_region-_an_overview_-_en_1.pdf.

[8] National Institute of Statistics. National Survey on Population and Housing 2009. Tunis. Cited by Economic and Social Commission of Western Asia (ESCWA) & League of Arab States. URL: https://www.unescwa.org/sites/www.unescwa.org/files/page_attachments/disability_in_the_arab_region-_an_overview_-_en_1.pdf.

[9] Gutenbrunner C, Nugraha B. Responding to the world health organization global disability action plan in Egypt: a technical consultation to develop a national disability health and rehabilitation plan. J Rehabil Med 2018;50(4):333-7.

[10] Rowerder B Disability inclusion: Topic guide. Birmingham, UK: GSDRC, University of Birmingham 2015. URL: http://opendocs.id.ac.uk/opendocs/handle/123456789/13783/DisabilityInclusion.pdf?sequence=1.

[11] Lkhouf N. Disability statistics from the 2014 Moroccan census. Haut-commissariaut au pian 2017. URL: https://unstats.un.org/unsd/demographic-social/meetings/2017/oman-disability-measurement-and-statistics/Session%206?Morocco.pdf.

[12] Trani JF, Bakhshi P, Lopez D, Gall F, Brown D. La situation socioéconomique des personnes en situation de handicap au Maroc et en Tunisie: inégalités, coût et stigmatisation - Socioeconomic situation of persons with disabilities in Morocco and Tunisia: Inequalities, cost and stigma. Eur J Disabil Res 2017;11:215–33.

[13] Hamed El Sahly RM, Cusick A. Rehabilitation services in Benghazi, Libya: An organizational case study. MEJFM 2016;14(9):11-18.

[14] Kanter AS, Sore I, Van Sant D. ‘Country Report: Tunisia. ADRY 2015;3:265-87. doi.org/10.17159/2413-7138/2015/v3n1a12.

[15] HI. Handicap International- information federale- Country card Algeria 2016. URL: https://handicap-international.de/sn_uploads/de/country/2016-08_cc_algeria_en_ok_0.pdf.

[16] Sida. Disability rights in the Middle East and North Africa 2014. URL: https://www.sida.se/globalassests/sida/eng/partners/human-rights-based-approach/disability/rights-of-persons-with-disabilities-mena.pdf.

[17] REACH. IDP protection monitoring assessment _ Libya. UNHCR 2016. URL: https://reliefweb.int/sites/reliefweb.int/files/resources/160322%20FINAL%20PAL%20Report.pdf.

[18] Trani JF, Bakhshi P, Tiapek S, Lopez D, Gall F. Disability and poverty in Morrocco and Tunisia: A multidimensional approach. J Hum. Dev Capab 2015;16(4):518-548.

[19] USDS. Sudan 2017 human rights report. United States Department of State 2017. URL: https://www.state.gov/documents/organization/277295.pdf.

[20] USDS. Tunisia 2017 human rights report. United States Department of State 2017. URL: https://www.state.gov/documents/organization/265734.pdf.

[21] African Studies and African Country Resources @ Pitt. North Africa Countries 2018. URL: https://pitt.libguides.com/c.php?g=123788p=65817.

[22] Institute on Disability. 2016 Disability Statistics Annual Report Rehabilitation Research and Training Centre on Disability Statistics and demographics 2017. URL: https://disabilitycompedium.org/sites/default/files/user-uploads/2016_AnnualReport.pdf.

[23] Office for Disability Issues and Department for Work and Pension. Disability prevalence estimates 2002/03 to 2011/12 Great Britain, 2012. URL: https://assets.publishing.service.gov.uk/government/uploads/system/uploads/attachment_data/file/321594/disability-prevalence.pdf.

[24] Adesina MA, Kanmodi KK. Prevalence and Socio-demographic distribution of people living with disability in the southern region of Africa. Adv Multidisc Sci Res J 2018 (Accepted).

[25] USDS. Equatorial Guinea 2016 human rights report. United States Department of State 2016. URL: https://www.state.gov/documents/organization/277239.pdf.

[26] Nord J. Disability statistics: an integral but missing (and misunderstood) component of development work. Hum Rights 2018;31(3):306-24.

[27] El Zawahry A. The effects of photovoice on explicit and implicit prejudice towards persons with disability. Master of Arts thesis in community psychology. The American University in Cairo 2018. URL: http://dar.aucegypt/bitstream/handle/10526/5230/Thesis%20final2018.TheEfffectsofPhotovoiceonPrejudicedocx.pdf?sequence=3.

SECTION TWO: ACKNOWLEDGMENTS

In: Disability: International Aspects
Editors: Ariel Tenenbaum et al.
ISBN: 978-1-53617-886-9

Chapter 16

ABOUT THE EDITORS

Ariel Tenenbaum, MD is the director of the Center for Children with Chronic Diseases at the Hadassah-Hebrew University Medical Center at the Mount Scopus Campus, Jerusalem, Israel. He graduated the Hadassah-Hebrew University Medical School and after pediatric residency at the Department of Pediatrics at Mount Scopus Campus, he continued his work at the hospital as a senior pediatric consultant and teacher of medical students. In 2004 he was appointed the head of the new Israeli Down syndrome program in the hospital. In 2005 he started the pre-adoption clinic together with Professor Isaiah D. Wexler. In 2012 he opened the Hadassah Intellectual and Developmental Disability Multidisciplinary Evaluation Center in collaboration with the Ministry of Social Affairs. He co-founded the Disability Studies Center at the Hebrew University, where he teaches students from humanities and social studies. He was recently appointed as a child development consultant. In 2019 he was elected to the Israeli Pediatric Association Committee and serves as its scientific secretary. His main research topics are disabilities, adoption, chronic diseases and general pediatrics. He has published numerous book chapters, edited several books, and published dozens of scientific articles in international journals. E-mail: tene@hadassah.org.il

Joav Merrick, MD, MMedSci, DMSc, born and educated in Denmark is professor of pediatrics, Division of Pediatrics, Hadassah Hebrew University Medical Center, Mt Scopus Campus, Jerusalem, Israel and Kentucky Children's Hospital, University of Kentucky, Lexington, Kentucky United States and professor of public health at the Center for Healthy Development, School of Public Health, Georgia State University, Atlanta, United States, the former medical director of the Health Services, Division for Intellectual and Developmental Disabilities, Ministry of Social Affairs and Social Services, Jerusalem, the founder and director of the National Institute of Child Health and Human Development in Israel. Numerous publications in the field of pediatrics, child health and human development, rehabilitation, intellectual disability, disability, health, welfare, abuse, advocacy, quality of life and prevention. Received the Peter Sabroe Child Award for outstanding work on behalf of Danish Children in 1985 and the International LEGO-Prize ("The Children's Nobel Prize") for an extraordinary contribution towards improvement in child welfare and well-being in 1987. In 2017 appointed a Kentucky Colonel by the Commonwealth of Kentucky, the highest honor the governor can bestow to a person. E-mail: jmerrick@zahav.net.il

In: Disability: International Aspects
Editors: Ariel Tenenbaum et al.
ISBN: 978-1-53617-886-9

Chapter 17

About the Center for Children with Chronic Diseases and Down Syndrome Center Jerusalem, Israel, Department of Pediatrics, Mt Scopus Campus, Hadassah Hebrew University Medical Center, Jerusalem, Israel

Chronic illnesses are common among children. These conditions last longer than a year and require continuous medical care and special needs. It is estimated that 10-20% of children in developed countries have one or more chronic condition. Advances in medicine and technology lead to an increase in the survival rate and longevity of children with chronic diseases and special needs. The severity of different chronic illnesses is variable, but there are many similarities. The child with a chronic illness faces physical, social, and emotional challenges. Therefore, medical care is not sufficient without rehabilitative service and emotional care for the child and his family.

Chronic illnesses are time and energy consuming. These children go through treatments, procedures and many healthcare visits. At home they often continue treatments as well, e.g., physiotherapy, breathing support machines and medications. This lifestyle may have detrimental effect on the child's social and emotional well-being, and similarly affect his parents and siblings.

Center for Children with Chronic Diseases

The aim of the Center for Children with Chronic Diseases at the Hadassah-Hebrew University Medical Center at the Mount Scopus Campus, Jerusalem, is to enhance medical care, comfort and well-being of patients and their families in the hospital and beyond. The center provides integrated and comprehensive care for these patients. This includes extensive support services and helping their families cope with the burden of care.

Numerous pediatric specialty programs and medical divisions have been established in the center to care for specific chronic conditions; among them are cystic fibrosis, Down syndrome, diabetes mellitus, familial dysautonomia, neuromuscular diseases, rheumatic diseases, feeding disorders and metabolic diseases. All these programs include evaluation and support from common services in the center: Nursing, nutrition, psycho-social care, speech therapy, physiotherapy and more.

The center works as a "one stop shop" for these children; As many services as possible, under one roof, on the same visit. Centralizing the care enables parents to come to one location to receive care. The physicians and nurses coordinate the care of the children thereby alleviating some of the burden of care off the families.

Children who are included in the programs of the center usually need returning visits to various medical specialists, consultations by multidisciplinary health professionals and performing diagnostic tests e.g., blood work, x-rays and respiratory functions. Some children may need hospitalization or palliative care. The center can concentrate all diagnostic and follow-up testing, medical surveillance and treatment in the hands of an experienced staff who knows the child and his unique situation.

The center is situated close to the entrance of the hospital and the families can access it without going through the main hospital building. In the center there are ten rooms for consultations. In addition, there are dedicated rooms for tests, e.g., respiratory functions, blood tests, sweat test and more. There is a large space with eight beds for continuous treatments, for example intravenous immunoglobulins and biological medications. In this space several unique tests are performed as well, for example growth hormone test and allergy challenge tests. There is also a special room for procedures, in which children can go through painful treatments with appropriate anesthetics and surveillance.

A special classroom in the center is operated by the ministry of education. In the classroom, children can continue their studies or play and interact with other children, in arts and crafts and many other programs.

The center is surrounded by a large healing garden that is partially maintained by the children themselves.

Conclusion

In conclusion, we believe that the "all inclusive" model of a center for children with chronic conditions is beneficial for the children and their families in terms of health and quality of life, and that this model is currently the best service for them.

Contact

Ariel Tenenbaum, MD, Isaiah D Wexler, MD, PhD
Center for Children with Chronic Diseases, Department of Pediatrics,
Mt Scopus Campus, Hadassah Hebrew University Medical Center,
Jerusalem, Israel
E-mail: TENE@hadassah.org.il

In: Disability: International Aspects
Editors: Ariel Tenenbaum et al.
ISBN: 978-1-53617-886-9

Chapter 18

About the National Institute of Child Health and Human Development in Israel

The National Institute of Child Health and Human Development (NICHD) in Israel was established in 1998 as a virtual institute under the auspices of the Medical Director, Ministry of Social Affairs and Social Services in order to function as the research arm for the Office of the Medical Director. In 1998 the National Council for Child Health and Pediatrics, Ministry of Health and in 1999 the Director General and Deputy Director General of the Ministry of Health endorsed the establishment of the NICHD.

Mission

The mission of a National Institute for Child Health and Human Development in Israel is to provide an academic focal point for the scholarly interdisciplinary study of child life, health, public health, welfare, disability, rehabilitation, intellectual disability and related aspects of human development. This mission includes research, teaching, clinical work, information and public service activities in the field of child health and human development.

SERVICE AND ACADEMIC ACTIVITIES

Over the years many activities became focused in the south of Israel due to collaboration with various professionals at the Faculty of Health Sciences (FOHS) at the Ben Gurion University of the Negev (BGU). Since 2000 an affiliation with the Zusman Child Development Center at the Pediatric Division of Soroka University Medical Center has resulted in collaboration around the establishment of the Down Syndrome Clinic at that center. In 2002 a full course on "Disability" was established at the Recanati School for Allied Professions in the Community, FOHS, BGU and in 2005 collaboration was started with the Primary Care Unit of the faculty and disability became part of the master of public health course on "Children and society". In the academic year 2005-2006 a one semester course on "Aging with disability" was started as part of the master of science program in gerontology in our collaboration with the Center for Multidisciplinary Research in Aging. In 2010 collaborations with the Division of Pediatrics, Hadassah Hebrew University Medical Center, Jerusalem, Israel around the National Down Syndrome Center and teaching students and residents about intellectual and developmental disabilities as part of their training at this campus.

RESEARCH ACTIVITIES

The affiliated staff have over the years published work from projects and research activities in this national and international collaboration. In the year 2000 the International Journal of Adolescent Medicine and Health and in 2005 the International Journal on Disability and Human Development of De Gruyter Publishing House (Berlin and New York) were affiliated with the National Institute of Child Health and Human Development. From 2008 also the International Journal of Child Health and Human Development (Nova Science, New York), the International Journal of Child and Adolescent Health (Nova Science) and the Journal of Pain Management (Nova Science) affiliated and from 2009 the International Public Health Journal (Nova Science) and Journal of Alternative Medicine Research (Nova Science). All peer-reviewed international journals.

NATIONAL COLLABORATIONS

Nationally the NICHD works in collaboration with the Faculty of Health Sciences, Ben Gurion University of the Negev; Department of Physical Therapy, Sackler School of Medicine, Tel Aviv University; Autism Center, Assaf HaRofeh Medical Center; National Rett and PKU Centers at Chaim Sheba Medical Center, Tel HaShomer; Department of Physiotherapy, Haifa University; Department of Education, Bar Ilan University, Ramat Gan, Faculty of Social Sciences and Health Sciences; College of Judea and Samaria in Ariel and in 2011 affiliation with Center for Pediatric Chronic Diseases and National Center for Down Syndrome, Department of Pediatrics, Hadassah Hebrew University Medical Center, Mount Scopus Campus, Jerusalem.

INTERNATIONAL COLLABORATIONS

Internationally with the Department of Disability and Human Development, College of Applied Health Sciences, University of Illinois at Chicago; Strong Center for Developmental Disabilities, Golisano Children's Hospital at Strong, University of Rochester School of Medicine and Dentistry, New York; Centre on Intellectual Disabilities, University of Albany, New York; Centre for Chronic Disease Prevention and Control, Health Canada, Ottawa; Chandler Medical Center and Children's Hospital,

Kentucky Children's Hospital, Section of Adolescent Medicine, University of Kentucky, Lexington; Chronic Disease Prevention and Control Research Center, Baylor College of Medicine, Houston, Texas; Division of Neuroscience, Department of Psychiatry, Columbia University, New York; Institute for the Study of Disadvantage and Disability, Atlanta; Center for Autism and Related Disorders, Department Psychiatry, Children's Hospital Boston, Boston; Department of Pediatric and Adolescent Medicine, Western Michigan University Homer Stryker MD School of Medicine, Kalamazoo, Michigan, United States; Department of Paediatrics, Child Health and Adolescent Medicine, Children's Hospital at Westmead, Westmead, Australia; International Centre for the Study of Occupational and Mental Health, Düsseldorf, Germany; Centre for Advanced Studies in Nursing, Department of General Practice and Primary Care, University of Aberdeen, Aberdeen, United Kingdom; Quality of Life Research Center, Copenhagen, Denmark; Nordic School of Public Health, Gottenburg, Sweden, Scandinavian Institute of Quality of Working Life, Oslo, Norway; The Department of Applied Social Sciences (APSS) of The Hong Kong Polytechnic University Hong Kong.

Targets

Our focus is on research, international collaborations, clinical work, teaching and policy in health, disability and human development and to establish the NICHD as a permanent institute in Israel in order to conduct model research.

Contact

Professor Joav Merrick, MD, MMedSci, DMSc
National Institute of Child Health and Human Development,
Jerusalem, Israel.
E-mail: jmerrick@zahav.net.il

SECTION THREE: INDEX

INDEX

A

F

G

H

I

Q

R

S

T

U

V

W

Y

Z